RELIGION AND HEALTHCARE

RELIGION AND SPIRITUALITY

Additional books in this series can be found on Nova's website under the Series tab.

Additional E-books in this series can be found on Nova's website under the E-books tab.

HEALTH CARE ISSUES, COSTS AND ACCESS

Additional books in this series can be found on Nova's website under the Series tab.

Additional E-books in this series can be found on Nova's website under the E-books tab.

RELIGION AND SPIRITUALITY

RELIGION AND HEALTHCARE

ANTHONY M. CURTIS
AND
DANIELLE P. WERTHEL
EDITORS

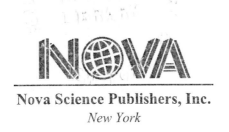

Nova Science Publishers, Inc.
New York

Copyright © 2012 by Nova Science Publishers, Inc.

For permission to use material from this book please contact us:
Telephone 631-231-7269; Fax 631-231-8175
Web Site: http://www.novapublishers.com

NOTICE TO THE READER

The Publisher has taken reasonable care in the preparation of this book, but makes no expressed or implied warranty of any kind and assumes no responsibility for any errors or omissions. No liability is assumed for incidental or consequential damages in connection with or arising out of information contained in this book. The Publisher shall not be liable for any special, consequential, or exemplary damages resulting, in whole or in part, from the readers' use of, or reliance upon, this material. Any parts of this book based on government reports are so indicated and copyright is claimed for those parts to the extent applicable to compilations of such works.

Independent verification should be sought for any data, advice or recommendations contained in this book. In addition, no responsibility is assumed by the publisher for any injury and/or damage to persons or property arising from any methods, products, instructions, ideas or otherwise contained in this publication.

This publication is designed to provide accurate and authoritative information with regard to the subject matter covered herein. It is sold with the clear understanding that the Publisher is not engaged in rendering legal or any other professional services. If legal or any other expert assistance is required, the services of a competent person should be sought. FROM A DECLARATION OF PARTICIPANTS JOINTLY ADOPTED BY A COMMITTEE OF THE AMERICAN BAR ASSOCIATION AND A COMMITTEE OF PUBLISHERS.

Additional color graphics may be available in the e-book version of this book.

Library of Congress Cataloging-in-Publication Data

Religion and healthcare / editors, Anthony M. Curtis and Danielle P. Werthel.
     p. cm.
   Includes index.
   ISBN 978-1-61324-256-8 (hardcover)
   1. Medical care--Religious aspects. 2. Care of the sick--Religious aspects. I. Curtis, Anthony M. II. Werthel, Danielle P.
   BL65.M4R4375 2011
   201'.7621--dc22
                                2011009080

Published by Nova Science Publishers, Inc. †New York

CONTENTS

PREFACE

This new book presents current research in the study of the relationship between religion and health care. Topics discussed include distributive justice and Christian health care ethics; hospitalized patients' expectations of spiritual care from nurses; faith-based substance abuse treatment programs; spiritual coping among chronically ill children and implications of integrative health care in religion.

Chapter 1 - A review of the literature shows that the closest approximation to a model which reflects the Christian principle of distributive justice in allocation and distribution of limited health care resources is that provided by Zoloth, who discusses four theories of justice. However, none of the four theories of distributive justice fully satisfy the theory of Christian theistic ethics. Most models reflect only rationales for increasing the amounts of resources available rather than allocating scarce resources. Using the summum bonum of the Ten Commandments, the author proposes a model which attempts to allocate scarce resources on the basis of distributive justice

Chapter 2 - Nurses are aware that the profession of nursing is holistic, that every action taken in the care of a patient has consequences, and they like to believe that those consequences have a positive impact on the patient and their family's ultimate health. For nurses, gaining an understanding of patients' expectations regarding spiritual care is essential to entering into a truly holistic, caring relationship with patients. The purpose of this phenomenological study was to explore the expectations patients have of nurses and how patients describe good nursing care. Specifically, questions were posed to reveal participants' perceptions of spiritual care provided by their nurses. Using Paterson's and Zderad's framework of humanistic nursing, 11 participants were interviewed. Data were analyzed using the Giorgi method of repetitive reflection. Findings suggested that participants appreciated nursing presence, being there, as having a positive influence on their health and well being, and elements of nursing presence were used to describe good nursing care. In fact, the spiritual element of nursing presence, being with, comprised the most defining characteristics of good nursing care, but, paradoxically, was not expected. Sharing of self by nurses was appreciated from the participants' perspective. All participants were able to define spirituality, most frequently in terms of religiosity; and religious elements of spirituality were not expected, nor welcomed, by most participants. Participants revealed that they perceived nurses to be busy, and this perceived lack of time was offered as a rationale for not expecting spiritual care.

Chapter 3 – One of the most troubling and persistent challenges in the field of psychology is the gulf between research and practice. Greenberg (1994) laments, "the two groups are separated virtually from professional birth" (p. 1). This estrangement has various consequences, ranging from a major split within the American Psychological Association (APA)—resulting in the formation of the American Psychological Society (APS)—to disputes about the practical relevance of empirically validated treatment procedures.

Chapter 4 - Children with chronic and potentially life-threatening illnesses are confronted with numerous stressors. Fear and uncertainty regarding the future, unpredictable illness course and outcome, intrusive treatment regimens, invasive medical procedures, perceived or actual loss of control, and general disruption of life events are a few of the many challenges they must face. Numerous studies conducted with chronically ill children support the idea of tailoring treatment to the individual needs of the patient by assessing developmental, familial, and cultural influences. Yet, surprisingly there has been relatively little attention paid in research to the manner in which children use religion/spirituality to help them through these stresses of chronic illness. Adult studies have clearly indicated that many people report turning to their faith beliefs when faced with a crisis such as an illness or an injury. While research on religious/spiritual coping in adults is enjoying growing interest, religious/spiritual coping in children has largely been neglected.

This chapter will review and discuss existing theories and research on children's spiritual coping, specifically as it pertains to dealing with chronic childhood illness. Clinical implications in the field of pediatric psychology and directions for future research in this area will also be explored.

Chapter 5 - The movement to integrate complementary and alternative medical (CAM) therapies—such as acupuncture and traditional oriental medicine, chiropractic, massage therapy, and herbal medicine—into conventional health care is replete with social, ethical, institutional, and legal challenges. Overall, inclusion of CAM therapies represents a historical shift from biomedical dominance to a more inclusive, pluralistic, and holistic method of care, one that explicitly acknowledges value in healing traditions other than that variously known as "conventional care" or "biomedicine." But this movement—broadly known in some circles as "integrative medicine" (or integrative health care)—has even deeper implications than achieving a fuller range of health care choices and a more holistic model of health. Notably, with its explicit emphasis on medical pluralism, integrative health care gives voice to a broad range of healing traditions and thus weaves in insights about human health and healing from other disciplines. In particular, therapies relying on human consciousness and intentionality (for example, prayer, visualization, and mental healing) can be seen to lie at the "borderland of healing and medicine," and thus, in the quest for understanding, to call for participation of sociologists, transpersonal psychologists, scholars of religion, and allied disciplines within the humanities. This chapter explores in preliminary form some of these links between integrative health care and religion, psychology and the humanities.

In: Religion and Healthcare   ISBN 978-1-61324-256-8
Editors: A.M. Curtis and D.P. Werthel   © 2012 Nova Science Publishers, Inc.

Chapter 1

DISTRIBUTIVE JUSTICE AND CHRISTIAN HEALTH CARE ETHICS: A PROPOSED MODEL BASED ON A REVIEW OF THE LITERATURE

*Marc D. Wooten**

ABSTRACT

A review of the literature shows that the closest approximation to a model which reflects the Christian principle of distributive justice in allocation and distribution of limited health care resources is that provided by Zoloth, who discusses four theories of justice. However, none of the four theories of distributive justice fully satisfy the theory of Christian theistic ethics. Most models reflect only rationales for increasing the amounts of resources available rather than allocating scarce resources. Using the summum bonum of the Ten Commandments, the author proposes a model which attempts to allocate scarce resources on the basis of distributive justice.

* Corresponding author: 915 Calverton Court, Fort Wayne, Indiana 46825, Phone: 260-426-5431 x71245, Fax: 260-426-5431 x17251, E-mail: mwooten1@juno.com.

I. PROLOGUE

Justice is a virtue that determines the proper limits and applications of intervening power.[1] Distributive justice is defined as the form of justice "which specifies a fair allocation of a society's wealth, resources, and power."[2] Buijsen traces justice in health care to the Roman legal maxim, "to each his own," or to each according to his need.[3] The Christian worldview on providing health care most clearly emanates from the sixth commandment not to kill (a negative deontological command). Amplifying this command is the parable of the good Samaritan, wherein the Samaritan was commended for providing benevolence in the form health care for the man attacked on the road to Jericho (Luke 10:25-37). Ultimately the obligation to provide health care derives its force from Jesus Christ's summation of one of the two great commandments, "to love one's neighbor as oneself," (Luke 10:27 [Leviticus 19:18], Matthew 22:39, Mark 12:31), which is also later repeated in the epistles (Romans 13:9, Galatians 5:14, James 2:8).

Furthermore, Jesus modeled compassion as He healed the sick, and also commissioned His disciples to do so (Matthew 4:23, 10:1, Luke 13:12). Caring for the sick is commended in Matthew 25:36 and James 5:14-15. Providing health care, then, draws from a perpetually binding commandment (the sixth), although the nuance of health care itself is a temporally binding command which will not be in view in the new earth (Revelation 21:4, 22:2-3). Healing the sick can also be traced back to the creation mandate for man to exercise dominion over the creation, although sickness itself came about as a result of the fall. Mott and Sider also argue that the drive for providing health care is based on the *imago Dei*, with a mutual obligation of all human beings for common good based on the fact that all persons possess that image.[4]

That one should look a distributive justice in health care at all is based on the recognition that resources are limited and need to be allocated. Some models such as the egalitarian model of justice have as an assumption that there is an unlimited supply of such resources. However, two drivers have been identified with increased consumption of health care resources. The first

---

[1] Stephen Mott and Ronald J. Sider, "Economic Justice: A Biblical Paradigm," in Art Beals and Larry Libby, eds., *Beyond Hunger: A Biblical Mandate for Social Responsibility* (Portland: Multnomah Press, 1985), 24.

[2] Ibid., 17.

[3] Martin Buijsen, "The Meaning of 'Justice' in Health Care," *Medicine and Law* 27.3 (2008):535-545.

[4] See note 1 above, p. 20.

is the argument that health care is in the category of necessities which could result in a life or death decision if they were denied. The second is that the advance of technology with more expensive and complex treatments became a matter of expensive communal pursuit. As a result, the desire of health care services has become not only an individual but a communal desire.[5] The result is an inequality between demand and supply of health care resources.

A fully developed model of distributive justice in health care would look at both the distribution of resources as well as the supply and demand that impact the resources that are available. However, most Christian critiques of distributive justice in health care deal solely with increasing the supply of health care dollars to purchase needed resources or limiting demand. For example, Cochran argues that that there is a need for further supply of money to enable purchase of these resources by the government to the poor.[6] Sider's proposals include both governmental solutions and expanded roles for Christian congregations and nonprofit organizations to provide health care to the poor.[7] Braun, speaking for The Hastings Center, attacks the demand for health care resources in her article regarding reprogenetics in Germany.[8] Rae, speaking for The Center for Bioethics and Human Dignity, correctly addresses the question of futility of care as it impacts demand for health care.[9]

In addition, supply and demand at the macrocosmic level can be looked at from both the deontological and consequential models (more frequently the latter than the former), as well as occasionally from the virtue model of obligation (when dealing with altruistic health care delivery systems such as in the third world). Despite the impact of adjustments caused by shifts in supply and demand at the macroscopic level, it is fair to assume that the sum of health care resources on a microcosmic level which are left to distribute in a given region or sector of American health care remains finite, if not relatively static.

Furthermore, Daniels points out that decisions regarding distribution at both the macro and micro level share three key features: (1) they are not

---

[5] Laurie Zoloth, *Health Care and the Ethics of Encounter: A Jewish Discussion of Social Justice* (Chapel Hill: University of North Carolina Press, 1999), 50-51.

[6] Clarke E. Cochran, "Health Policy and the Poverty Trap," in Art Beals and Larry Libby, eds., *Beyond Hunger: A Biblical Mandate for Social Responsibility* (Portland: Multnomah Press, 1985), 229-260.

[7] Ronald J. Sider, *Just Generosity: A New Vision for Overcoming Poverty in America* (Grand Rapids: Baker Books, 1999), 173-189.

[8] Kathrin Braun, "Not Just for Experts: The Public Debate about Reprogenetics in Germany," *The Hastings Center Report* 35.3 (2005):42-49.

[9] Scott B. Rae, "Money and Health Care in the New Millennium," http://www.cbhd. orgresources/ healthcare.rae_2000-10-12.htm. Accessed on 1/6/2009.

sufficiently divisible to avoid unequal distributions, (2) some people will be denied benefits even though they can claim that they have a plausible right to them in principle, and (3) the general distribution principles to which claimants appeal do not sufficiently discriminate between similar claimants.[10] Given the presumption of a finite amount of resources, this essay will examine the models of distribution of health care dollars without adjusting either supply or demand with the goal of determining the impact of Christian theistic ethics on these models. It is not assumed as a result of this discussion that God cannot, according to His sovereign plan, at any time choose to heal someone outside of the domain of established health care resources.

II. MODELS AND THEORIES OF DISTRIBUTIVE JUSTICE

There is no uniform agreement on the models or theories of distributive justice. Wolff identifies three models of distributive justice—justice as mutual advantage, justice as reciprocity, and justice as impartiality.[11] These correspond to Zoloth's description of four theories of justice. The first is the libertarian theory emphasizing liberty, personal property, and entitlement, and promoting Lockean principles for distribution (similar to Wolff's "justice as mutual advantage"). The second is the utilitarian theory, based on Mill's thought, which emphasizes the common fate of all men and is a consequentialist theory with happiness as the key value. The third is the deontological theory based on Rawls and Kant, which argues that allocation of goods is a matter of procedural rules (having the most analogy to Wolff's "justice of reciprocity" emphasizing proportionality). The fourth is the egalitarian theory (employed in Veatch's thought) emphasizing the need to protect the least advantaged because of the fundamental equality of all (similar to Wolff's "justice as impartiality"). Zoloth further identifies five material principles of justice—numerical equality, need, individual effort, social contribution, and merit.[12] Some of these are incorporated as values in others' utilitarian models. Leget and Hoedemaekers describe an additional

---

[10] Norman Daniels, "Four Unsolved Rationing Problems: A Challenge," *The Hastings Center Report* 24.4 (1994):27-29.

[11] Jonathan Wolff, "Models of Distributive Justice," *Novartis Foundation Symposium* 278 (2007):165-170.

[12] See note 5 above, pp. 73-93.

communitarian theory based on what society determines is necessary healthcare (which seems to be a modified form of deontology).[13]

Boylan describes five theories of distributive justice: (1) competition (in part parallel to Zoloth's libertarian theory); (2) aristocracy (to each according to his inherited status, no parallels with either Wolff or Zoloth); (3) capitalism (parallel to Wolff's "justice as mutual advantage" and in part to Zoloth's libertarian theory), (4) socialism (parallel to Wolff's "justice as reciprocity" and Zoloth's utilitarian theory), and (5) egalitarianism (parallel to Wolff's "justice as impartiality" and Zoloth's egalitarian theory). Boylan identifies as part of the compassionate model of distributive justice the principles of commitment to excellence, being a cooperative member of the community, meeting legitimate needs, and being economically responsible.[14]

There is further subdivision within two of the four theories mentioned by Zoloth. Savulescu subdivides consequentialism within utilitarianism into reasons-based consequentialism and opportunism. He argues for the former, and proposes two alternatives: (1) the priority view (satisfying those first whom individually there is most reason to save), and (2) the additive view (giving some weight to less rational claims and summing these claims together prior to making a decision).[15] Hsu further points to the emotive component (presumably happiness) in distributive justice as a value for consequentialists.[16]

Fox further subdivides egalitarianism into four classes: (1) flat equality, (2) luck egalitarianism, (3) prioritarianism, and (4) sufficientarianism. Flat equality redistributes resources from the more well-off to the less well-off (a form of socialism). Luck egalitarianism holds individuals at least partially morally responsible for their need for health care (for example, sexually transmitted diseases). Prioritarianism gives preference to the least advantaged (Rawls) on the premise that greater benefit is derived from dividing up resources among the larger number of worse-off individuals than the smaller number of well-off individuals. Sufficientarianism is based in the premise that all individuals ought to be above some critical threshold of the currency of

[13] Carlo Leget and R. Hoedemaekers, "Teaching Medical Students About Fair Distribution of Healthcare Resources," *Journal of Medical Ethics* 33.12 (2007):737-741.

[14] Michael Boylan, "Medical Pharmaceuticals and Distributive Justice," *Cambridge Quarterly of Healthcare Ethics* 17.1 (2008):30-44.

[15] Julian Savulescu, "Consequentialism, Reasons, Value and Justice," *Bioethics* 12 (1998): 273-280.

[16] Ming Hsu, Cedric Anen, and Steven R. Quartz, "The Right and the Good: Distributive Justice and Neural Encoding of Equity and Efficiency," *Science* 320 (2008):1092-1095.

distribution.[17] Schramme takes the fourth category of Fox and combines a
naturalist theory of disease with a sufficientarianist model as a method for
allocating health care resources by arguing against treating dysfunctions for
which no disease has been proven (he does not specify what they are, but does
cite as an example a beef allergy for someone who is a vegetarian).[18]

The libertarian theory and the egalitarian theory have especially been the
focus of literature regarding models of distributive justice. The arguments used
to support the libertarian theory revert back to Zoloth's material principles of
merit, individual effort, and social contribution. For example, Havighurst and
Richman espouse a model which provides health care more generously for
those who pay more, and favor less governmental regulation. They argue that
the current system, for example, requires individuals to purchase more health
care (or better quality) than they can reasonably afford or will need.[19] Conover
contends that a disproportionate share of the costs of regulation is funneled to
the less well-off.[20] Others argue that health care decision making simply be
made more open and transparent to all parties involved, in line with the
libertarian theory.[21]

Zelenak, on the other hand, favors a taxation plan that falls more in line
with the egalitarian approach.[22] Miller maintains that normalization of health
care outcomes (an egalitarian ideal) would result in distributive justice.[23]
Hunter points the individual physician to a utilitarian/egalitarian discussion

[17] Dov Fox, "Luck, Genes, and Equality," *Journal of Law, Medicine, and Ethics* 35.4
(2007):716.

[18] Thomas Schramme, "The Significance of the Concept of Disease of Justice in Health
Care" *Theoretical Medicine and Bioethics* 28.2 (2007):121-135.

[19] Clark C. Havighurst and Barak D. Richman, "Distributive Injustice(s) in American
Health Care," *Law and Contemporary Problems* 69.4 (2006):7-81.

[20] Christopher J. Conover, "Distributive Considerations in the Overregulation of Health
Professionals, Health Facilities, and Health Plans," *Law and Contemporary Problems*
69.4 (2006):181-193.

[21] Mary Beth Foglia, et. al., "Priority Setting and the Ethics of Resource Allocation within
VA Healthcare Facilities: Results of a Survey," *Organizational Ethics* 4.2 (2008):83-96.

[22] Lawrence Zelenak, "Of Head Taxes, Income Taxes, and Distributive Justice in American
Health Care," *Law and Contemporary Problems* 69.4 (2006):103-120.

[23] Tom Miller, "Measuring Distributive Injustice on a Different Scale," *Law and
Contemporary Problems* 69.4 (2006):231-243.

with the patient.[24] Sreenivasan makes a case for international normatization of health care resources, thus arguing for international egalitarianism.[25]

In summary, Zoloth's four theories of distributive justice seem to be the best comprehensive framework for discussion of how to allocate scarce health care resources. Fox's fourfold segmentation of egalitarianism is the clearest way to understand this theory as it impacts health care.

III. CRITIQUE OF PROPOUNDED THEORIES AND MODELS

The Christian theistic model of ethics espouses the theory of obligation (the Ten Commandments), the properly basic beliefs (the *summum bonum* of the kingdom of God [Matthew 6:33]), and the theory of motivation. The role of the sixth commandment has been previously explained. The properly basic belief that the Christian is to live for and look for the kingdom of God drives the desire to see the destruction of evil in this world (physically as well as spiritually) as well as an ethic of hope looking forward to the day when the kingdom of God will destroy sin and its consequences (including sickness). Motivations which would impact health care would include compassion for the sick (as well as the poor), love, and service.

In view of these, the libertarian (Lockean/democratic) theory of distribution would meet the needs of some individuals but not others. Since the sixth command is a deontological command with a partial view to consequences, it would suggest that the libertarian view is not alone sufficient to distribute the health care resources in a closed system (particularly since the autonomy of the self is emphasized). Furthermore, the kingdom of God (the *summum bonum* of the New Testament) is not given to those with either their own resources or merit (Ephesians 2:8-9, 1 Corinthians 1:26-27), and therefore one would need to find other criteria than those two alone (which undergird the libertarian theory) to suffice to allocate resources. Lastly, it is possible that the motivations of the caregivers could extend to patients under the libertarian theory, but it prevents those same motivations from being extended to individuals who are less well-off. The *imago Dei* rests in all people, not just those who are well-off. Therefore, the libertarian theory of distributive justice

---

[24] David Hunter, "Am I my Brother's Gatekeeper? Professional Ethics and the Prioritization of Healthcare," *Journal of Medical Ethics* 33.9 (2007):522-526.

[25] Gopal Sreenivasan, "International Justice and Health: A Proposal," *Ethics and International Affairs* 16.2 (2002):81-90.

alone is not sufficient to account for distributive justice according to Christian theistic theory.

The consequentialist or utilitarian theory of distributive justice would assign all health care resources on the basis of the intrinsic value of happiness (or perhaps goodness). Since disease to the consequentialist represents the absence of happiness, resources should be assigned to eliminate the most unhappiness for the most people. Although the sixth commandment is deontological with a partial view toward consequences, the consequences in view do not appear to be maximization of happiness. Also, happiness is never in view as a value in the New Testament, but rather joy, and the *summum bonum* of the New Testament is to seek the kingdom of God (with the accompanying destruction of evil), not happiness.

Furthermore, this view assumes that there is no utilitarian value to disease. However, there is value in disease when it forces one to acknowledge the sovereignty of God and one's need for grace (2 Corinthians 12:9-10), when it is for the sake of the glory of God (John 9:3), and when it increases one's desire for the consummation of God's kingdom (Romans 8:19-25). Furthermore, disease can result in release to death (Hebrews 9:27), which is where those who believe in Christ experience ultimate victory over sin (1 Corinthians 15:54-57). The motivations of compassion, love, generosity, and service can all be used with or without respect to consequences. In addition, it is not always possible to restore the *imago Dei* through restoration of happiness. Therefore, the consequentialist theory of distributive justice seems not to have the support of Christian theistic ethics.

The egalitarian theory of distributive justice stresses the need to distribute all resources equally. Although the sixth commandment in its negative form is thoroughly egalitarian, in its positive restatement, neither the deontological nor the partial consequences components are satisfied by egalitarian distributive justice. While the Bible teaches one's responsibility towards one's neighbor (Matthew 22:39), it does not assume that all differences between individuals will be eliminated either outside of the kingdom of God or inside the kingdom. Fox's categories of luck egalitarianism and sufficientarianism at least hold people partially responsible for the choices that they have made, thus upholding some parts of the *imago Dei*.

The *summum bonum* of the New Testament, the kingdom of God, is represented in the parts of the egalitarian theory by the gift of grace made available towards those who do not deserve it and the ethic of hope based on the final destruction of evil. However, for some egalitarians this would lead to a world where the consummation of the kingdom is not necessary or even desirable. However, generosity (motivated by true humility) is one premise of the egalitarian theory which is taught in the New Testament (Matthew 25:36, James 2:8-9, 1 John 3:16-18). Therefore, while the egalitarian theory of distributive justice is not sufficient to account for distributive justice under Christian theistic ethics, it serves to offset the selfish nature of the libertarian theory of distributive justice.

The deontological theory of distributive justice presumes that there are dedicated principles for allocating health care resources. Given that the sixth commandment in its positive form is deontological with a partial view toward consequences, this suggests that this view at least partially satisfies Christian theistic ethics. The duty to preserve the *imago Dei* in the patient is preserved in this theory of distributive justice.

With regards to the *summum bonum* of the New Testament, the duty to deliver health care resources according to set principles may conflict with the grace which is to characterize the kingdom, particularly for those who must make the choices about where to distribute the resources. The duty to deliver health care according to set principles may also be overridden by the duty to seek God's kingdom, insofar as those called to spread that kingdom may find themselves subject to conditions of disease. Nevertheless, there remains for this theory the ethic of hope due to the final destruction of evil with the consummation of the kingdom of God. In the final analysis, the deontological theory of distributive justice at least partially satisfies Christian theistic ethics.

In summary, none of the four theories of distributive justice fully satisfy the theory of Christian theistic ethics. Of the four theories discussed, Jesus' actions with regard to healing the sick seem to come closest to a consequentialist (with a view to building their faith or leading them to faith in Him) or deontological (with a view to demonstrating His deity and sovereignty in establishing the kingdom by working miracles) theory. One critique of the use of Christ as an example, however, is that Jesus always healed people (He never just treated them). Hence, no principles were set out by Him as to who should be treated and who should not. Nevertheless, Jesus also identified with the sick.[26]

---

[26] See note 6 above, p. 234.

IV. A PROPOSED MODEL OF
HEALTH CARE DISTRIBUTION

Given that none of the four theories of distributive justice discussed above fully satisfy Christian theistic ethics, the *summum bonum* should be the starting point for developing a model of health care distribution which most fully satisfies the sixth commandment. Man's absolute state of perfection in the Garden of Eden was forfeited at the Fall, and this led to the corruption of the creation, including the introduction of sickness and disease. Since that time, man has relied on the gift of God's grace (both common and special) to help him overcome illness. Nonetheless, death has reigned from the first Adam until the consummation of the kingdom of God with the exception of Jesus' resurrection. Man therefore cooperates with God in being an instrument of that grace insofar as providing health care is concerned. The destruction of evil occurs when one chooses to repent and follow Christ and become a part of His kingdom. Health care may be used as an instrument to lead to that, as well as demonstrating God's common grace toward men by allowing partial or full recovery from illness, resulting in restoration to the community.[27] The ethic of hope is established by the expectation that at the consummation there will be no more sin and thus no more illness, with the full restoration of the creation.

One of the problems with the concept of justice in health care is that, when one has a disease, more often than not he/she does not desire justice, but rather mercy (in consonance with the second principle of the *summum bonum*. Since Christians are called to be people of mercy, the model must allow for allocation in part based on this principle. Likewise, the model should take into account God's special concern for the poor, as well as widows and orphans.[28]

Figure 1 represents a model for this allocation. The model first allows for the questions of eligibility (dealing with the question of "insurance" or whatever principle is used to ascertain that the patient is included in the class of individuals who may rightfully be treated) and the question of futility (whether a given treatment simply postpones death rather than prolonging life), both of which are deontological questions. The decision not to treat on the basis of futility should always be followed by an offer of palliative care. What follows next is the question of medical necessity, which is a consequentialist question. A large of number of treatments are not medically necessary (such as experimental therapies with no known benefit, sex change

---

[27] See note 1 above, p. 27.

[28] See note 1 above, p. 27.

operations, facial plastic surgery, or breast augmentation; one could include therapeutic abortion of pregnancy as well). A denial of these therapies would be accompanied by an explanation to the patient about the lack of medical necessity associated with these.

Having passed these questions, the decision-making process should be guided by Grushkin and Daniel's questions regarding accountability for reasonableness. Four conditions are mentioned for establishing such accountability: (1) the publicity condition (that rationales for decisions should be publically accessible); (2) the relevance condition (that rationales for decisions should be accompanied by a reasonable explanation); (3) the revision and appeals condition (that rationales for decisions may be challenged, with opportunity to change them in the light of new or better evidence); and (4) the regulative condition (that there is public regulation of the preceding three conditions to assure that they are met).[29]

Once these are satisfied, one additional question should be asked, which is whether or not the treatment can be provided by the body of Christ. The body should become proactive in the delivery of health care as part of its call to minister to a lost world. If such treatment is not available after satisfying these conditions, then the model would allow for the treatment to be given as long as resources are available in a given health care setting (a nod to Schramme's model of sufficientarianism/egalitarianism).

In conclusion, such a model would provide a deontological and consequentialist approach to distributive justice. Those who belong to the kingdom of God would be involved at all steps of the process, particularly in developing Daniels' accountability for reasonableness criteria. Their involvement as those who deliver the health care is crucial, with a need for the church to expand its role.

---

[29] Sofia Gruskin and Normal Daniels, "Justice and Human Rights: Priority Setting and Fair Deliberative Process," *American Journal of Public Health* 98.9 (2008):1573-1577.

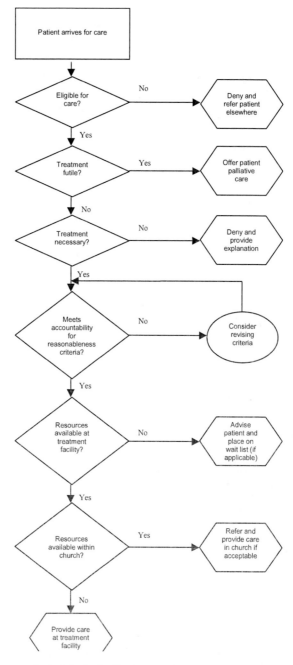

Figure 1. A Proposed Model of Distributive Justice.

In: Religion and Healthcare   ISBN 978-1-61324-256-8
Editors: A.M. Curtis and D.P. Werthel   © 2012 Nova Science Publishers, Inc.

Chapter 2

HOSPITALIZED PATIENTS' EXPECTATIONS OF SPIRITUAL CARE FROM NURSES

Lisa A. Davis
West Texas AandM University, Texas, U.S.A.

ABSTRACT

Nurses are aware that the profession of nursing is holistic, that every action taken in the care of a patient has consequences, and they like to believe that those consequences have a positive impact on the patient and their family's ultimate health. For nurses, gaining an understanding of patients' expectations regarding spiritual care is essential to entering into a truly holistic, caring relationship with patients. The purpose of this phenomenolo-gical study was to explore the expectations patients have of nurses and how patients describe good nursing care. Specifically, questions were posed to reveal participants' perceptions of spiritual care provided by their nurses. Using Paterson's and Zderad's framework of humanistic nursing, 11 participants were interviewed. Data were analyzed using the Giorgi method of repetitive reflection. Findings suggested that participants appreciated nursing presence, being there, as having a positive influence on their health and well being, and elements of nursing presence were used to describe good nursing care. In fact, the spiritual element of nursing presence, being with, comprised the most defining characteristics of good nursing care, but, paradoxically, was not expected. Sharing of self by nurses was appreciated from the participants' perspective. All participants were able to define spirituality, most frequently in terms of religiosity; and religious elements of spirituality were not expected, nor welcomed, by most participants. Participants revealed that they perceived nurses to be busy, and this perceived lack of time was offered as a rationale for not expecting spiritual care.

INTRODUCTION

The hallmark of nursing as a profession is that of holism, a concern with not only the physical health of the client, but the mental and spiritual health as well (Burkhart, 1989; Carson, 1989; Dossey, 1998; Fontaine, 2000; Patterson and Zderad, 1988; Stuart, Deckro, and Mandle, 1989; Taylor, 2002; Travelbee, 1969; Watson, 1999). Furthermore, nursing care should address needs that may arise from these human dimensions of body, mind and spirit and recognize the impact that each dimension has on the others (Patterson, 1998; Taylor, 2002). Martha Rogers (1972) further stipulated that the mind, body and spirit are an irreducible whole, not to be treated separately, and all (mind, body and spirit) contribute to overall human health with dynamic interplay.

Watson (1999) recognized holism in her assertion that persons need to be cared for and to find harmony in life. Given that, nursing is charged with helping people gain " a higher degree of harmony within the mind, body and soul" (Watson, 1999, p. 10). Dossey (1998) stresses that not focusing clinical attention to the concepts of mind, body and spirit in patient care is unscientific. Attention to issues of values and purpose in life are just as important as attention to physical parameters such as blood pressure. According to Benner (1985), nurses cannot understand health and illness by merely studying the mind or the body, but rather by studying the person in context. The integrality of body, mind, and spirit is central to holistic practice, so much so, that Quinn (2000) refers to the dimensions as bodymindspirit. Watson and Smith's (2002) framework of transpersonal caring emphasizes the spiritual dimension by honoring both nurse and patient as embodied spirits. Indeed, Bensley (1991) suggests that not only are body, mind and spirit dimensions of health, the spiritual dimension is the coordinator, the element that unifies the other dimensions of health. There is considerable discussion in nursing literature of the relative value of the dimensions of holism, but it is clear that value is placed in the holistic care of patients. Yet, nurses report they rarely, if ever, provide spiritual care (Stranahan, 2001; Thomas et al, 2002). The questions then arise: Are nurses meeting the needs of patients? Are those needs perceived as being met by patients?

PURPOSE OF STUDY

Nurses understand that while each person is a unique individual and responds individually to care, all humans are more alike than different and value comes from that common humanness (Patterson and Zderad, 1985). The purpose of this study was to explore the expectations patients have of nurses regarding the spiritual dimension of care and to identify how patients describe good nursing care. Philosophically, separating the spiritual dimension from the whole changes it. David Bohm (1996) refers to this as fragmentation – thought that divides. While the spiritual dimension is the concept of interest, it should be remembered that spirituality is part of a greater whole. As with dialogue, separation from the whole should not take on great importance. Rather, exploring the dimensions and understanding the integrality of the human experience is the ultimate goal. Nursing literature is replete with studies of nurses' perceptions of the meanings and constituents of spiritual care, while studies of patient perceptions of the meaning of spiritual care are few.

RATIONALE FOR THE STUDY

Nurses are aware that every action taken in the care of a patient has consequences and like to believe that those consequences have a positive impact on the patient and their family's ultimate health. Nursing actions such as administering blood products, clinical decision-making, and compassion are executed and have meaning to the nurse, but understanding is not achieved by singular experience. A caring relationship requires mutual understanding. Establishing a relationship is much like maintaining a dialog. As indicated by Bohm (1996), dialog is more than an effort at exchanging knowledge in order to have common information, but rather so that two people are making something *in common* (p. 2). Just as having a knowledge base and speaking without acknowledging the listener and what he/she has to say is incomplete, establishing care without the acknowledgement and participation of the patient is not a fully developed relationship. Understanding patients' perceptions regarding the spiritual care they receive and the spiritual care they expect can enhance the caring relationship, and in so doing, add to the overall understanding of the human condition and the impact that nursing has on the overall health of patients who find themselves in nursing's care.

After reviewing spiritual care and caring, there existed a gap in understanding the essence of patient expectations regarding the spiritual dimension of nursing care. For nurses, gaining that understanding is essential to entering into a truly holistic caring relationship with patients. There were four research questions pertinent to the purpose of this study (Davis, 2005):

1. Are the explicit and implicit actions of nurses to address body, mind and spirit recognized by patients?
2. Are the actions of nurses to address spiritual health perceived by patients as fulfilling a patient expectation?
3. What actions by nurses are perceived as spiritual interventions by patients?
4. How do individuals define spiritual care?

THEORETICAL FRAMEWORK

Nursing has a humanistic orientation, and the humanistic values are manifested in the artistic aspects of caring (Watson, 1985). Cumbie (2001) interprets humanistic nursing as more than the technically competent subject-object relationship of nurse to patient in which the nurse directs care for the benefit of the patient. Humanistic nursing involves more of a transaction between nurse and patient in which the nurse is cognizant of self and others through reflection on personal experiences. These various personal experiences allow the nurse to see the patient as more than a person with a medical diagnosis. A key element in humanistic nursing is the idea of presence; being open or available in a manner that the patient finds meaningful or comforting (Godkin, 2001); both 'being there' and 'being with' the patient (Patterson and Zderad, 1988; Nelms, 1996). As a result, the nurse and patient develop a trusting relationship that allows for the multidimensionality of nursing care.

Humanistic nursing (Patterson and Zderad, 1988) is concerned with the uniqueness of each human being. Each human being has a specific and individual history and experience, as well as a collective history and experience as a member of a community. Each human being has a different response to self, others and environment. Each human has value and perceives value in others. Therefore, human potential as well as human limitations are reflected by both the patient and the nurse. Both the nurse and the patient contribute to and gain from the relationship (Watson, 1985; Patterson and Zderad, 1988). Because the nurse-patient relationship is both transactional and interactional, both the nurse and the patient should perceive this existential quality.

Humanistic nursing is described in terms of being a dialogic phenomenon (Patterson and Zderad, 1988). It is expected that the nurse will be helpful to the patient in that the nurse actively attempts to meet the patient's needs. The patient then expects to be helped; to have needs met. The nurse is actively listening, observing, and assessing, and the patient is conveying cues, both verbally and nonverbally. However, the nurse and patient may differ in their perceptions of what those needs might be, how to meet them, and if, indeed, the needs have been met. Furthermore, that relationship can only be established when each participant, the nurse and the patient, perceive each other as unique individuals.

Although widely accepted, there is no consensus about the value of humanism as a framework for nursing and it has also been suggested that practicing humanistic care places the patient solely responsible for setting health care goals, thereby relieving the nurse from accountability for quality patient care (McKinnon, 1991). However, Travelbee (1969) suggested that establishing, maintaining and terminating the nurse patient relationship is the responsibility of the nurse. Moreover, McKinnon believes that humanistic nurses de-emphasize physical care and questions whether responsible choices can be made by the patient. Finally, being more subjective than objective, McKinnon believes that humanistic nursing theory does not attempt to validate the nursing process. This interpretation of humanism argues that humanism is not objective and therefore cannot be measured. True, humanism lends itself to phenomenologic study.

Because much of the nursing literature is vague, idealistic and inconsistent in applied definitions, Mulholland (1994) believes that the humanistic framework is inadequate to fully explicate the social, economic and political dynamics of the nurse-patient relationship. However, Mulholland believes the imprecise nature of humanism's ambiguity to be problematic rather than an outright indictment of humanism, suggesting more discourse on the ontologic and epistemologic foundations of humanism. This suggestion is certainly well-founded, nevertheless, I believed that, rather than a weakness, the strength of humanism as a framework was that the basis of humanism is not linearly prescriptive.

Phenomenology is a qualitative research methodology as well as a philosophical framework designed to explore human experiences from the standpoint of the everyday meaning ascribed to the lived experience by the individuals who experience them rather than theoretical meaning ascribed by an observer (Streubert and Carpenter, 1999; Van Mannen, 1990). Philosophically, phenomenology allows individuals to give voice to actual lived experiences and to their own beliefs and ideas to another individual with the intent of understanding the meaning of that lived experience. Meaning is found in the existential dialogic interplay between nurse and patient (Patterson and Zderad, 1988). Examining the implications of their meanings leads to better understanding of the phenomenon in question (Polkinghorne, 1988). The value of the dialogic experience is in its uniqueness. Each interplay between nurse and patient is important in developing the overall meaning of the experience. Patterson and Zderad (1988) espoused a necessity for a phenomenologic approach in humanistic nursing. Humanism encompasses:

> ...not a simple cataloguing of qualities or counting of elements...it involves an openness to nursing phenomena, a spirit of receptivity, readiness for surprise, the courage to experience the unknown...This being-with (subjective, intuitive knowing and experiencing) and looking at (objective analyzing) the phenomenon all at once sparks a creative synthesis, a conceptualization from which emanates insightful description (p. 79).

Phenomenology is a description of an experience based on the ideas, beliefs, knowledge and context of the moment. These internal and external factors do not remain constant. Time or subsequent life events may color the individual's perceptions of an event. The complexity of intrinsic and extrinsic factors will always exist, therefore alternate descriptions of an event will always exist (Van der Zalm and Bergum, 2000). Because of the possibility of a multiplicity of perceptions, it is not possible to assign inference or meaning, or to explain the events of the lived experience of another, but the recounting of the event, one to another, the "being with" and intuitive knowing as described by Patterson and Zderad are important in the discovery process.

Van Manen (1990) states that phenomenology is a study of essences. The essence is revealed by studying the details of the events of lived experience. Van Manen adds that, from the phenomenological perspective, the facts of the lived experience are less important than the essence of the experience (what was it like, rather than what was). "The essence or nature of an experience has been adequately described in language if the description reawakens or shows us the lived quality and significance of the experience in a fuller or deeper manner"(p.10).

ASSUMPTIONS

For purposes of this study, it was assumed that:

1. Nursing is holistic, therefore concerned with the overall health and well being of the patient, to include physical, mental and spiritual dimensions.
2. Spirituality is a dimension of health.
3. Health is not defined by physical, mental or spiritual well-being, but by the dynamic juxtaposition of each on the other.
4. Participants in the study will respond honestly.

REVIEW OF THE LITERATURE

Spirituality and purpose in life have been studied in conjunction with other concepts such as quality of life, stressful life events, general health, depression, death acceptance, goal seeking and religious orientation. The main source of literature for the constructs included professional journals in nursing, theology, psychology, occupational health, and sociology. Spirituality as an element of holism is accepted in nursing. There is a lack of consensus regarding the definition of spirituality, however, discovering purpose or meaning in life is a central issue of spirituality. A theoretical exploration of the concepts of holism, spirituality, purpose in life, caring, and spiritual care are presented. Second, quantitative studies related to aspects of spirituality are explored. Lastly, qualitative studies regarding patient satisfaction, patient expectations regarding spirituality and caring in general are considered.

Central to holistic care are spirituality and healing which L. Dossey and B. Dossey (1998) state "encompass a person's values, meaning and purpose in life. They reflect the human traits of caring, love, honesty, wisdom and imagination and they may reflect belief in a higher power, higher existence or a guiding spirit" (p. 46). Because nursing is holistic, it is problematic that descriptions of the components of spirituality are quite diverse, with little consensus toward meaning (Carson, 1989; Taylor, 2002). The intangible nature of spirituality is compounded by the reality that it is shaped by cultural components as well as the context in which it is interpreted. There is a challenge for nursing to define spirituality in such a way as to take into account the importance and relevance of the dimension of spirituality without it being taken out of context or losing clarity with regard to nursing (McSherry and Draper, 1998).

The root of the word, spirit is from Latin meaning "breathe" (Woolf, 1978). As both fundamental and essential as the act of breathing, Carson (1989) asserts that spirituality is what defines us all as unique individuals. Taylor (2002) defines spirituality as "an innate, universal aspect of being human ...[that] integrates, motivates, energizes and influences every aspect of a person's life (p. 5)." Goldberg (1998) identifies concepts such as meaning, presence, empathy, compassion, hope, love, religion, transcendence, touch and healing as aspects of spirituality important to nursing (as cited in Taylor, 2002). Davidhizar, Bechtel and Cosey (2000) add that the nursing intervention of presence, both "being there" in the physical sense and "being with" in the psychological and spiritual sense is the most essential nursing intervention.

Patients, when faced with illness, often question the fundamental meaning of their lives. A sense of purpose in life has been identified as the seminal indicator or outcome of spiritual health (Carson et al, 1992; Frankl, 1984). Frankl observed that purpose of life was a unique trait that had to be identified and fulfilled by each person individually.

Travelbee (1968) asserts that nursing is an interpersonal process in which the role of the nurse is to help the individual/family to find meaning in illness experiences. As did Frankl, Travelbee believed that humans are motivated by meaning, and the illness experience offers a unique opportunity for the nurse to both witness and assist the ill person and the family to discover meaning. Newman (1989) also acknowledges the interpersonal process, stating that human interaction is a spiritual component. It is unclear from the literature whether spiritual growth allows one to know his/her purpose in life or if purpose in life is what allows spiritual growth, but the two are inextricably intertwined.

Wright (1998) defines spirituality as that "dimension of a person that involves one's relationship with self, other, the natural order, and a higher power manifested through creative expressions, familiar rituals, meaningful work, and religious practices" (p.81). Espland (1999) adds that spiritual wellness is that part of the individual that gives purpose to life. Further, a lack of meaning can lead to spiritual distress, hopelessness and despair. Purpose in life involves a search for relationships and situations that provide a sense of worth and a reason for living.

Richards (1991) identifies faith as a belief system that helps the individual develop a purpose in life. However, spirituality is a broader concept than religion (O'Neill and Kenny, 1998; Sheldon, 2000). It may or may not incorporate religious rituals. In fact, nonreligious or atheistic individuals have the spiritual need to find meaning or purpose in life (Tanyi, 2002). Reed (1987) defined spirituality in terms of values and behaviors that relate to something greater than self. In addition, she identifies indicators of spirituality as engaging in prayer, having a meaning to life, contemplation, closeness to a higher being, sense of community and a sense of awareness. Ross (1994) identifies aspects of spirituality as being: purpose and fulfillment, hope or will to live, and faith in self, others and God. B. Howard and J. Howard (1996) suggest that one's occupation is a spiritual activity, stating that how individuals spend their time is a crucial part of their well-being. Prayer and meaning or purpose in life are identified as empirical indicators for appraising spirituality (Meraviglia, 1999).

Burkhart (1989) describes spirituality as a process and a sacred journey to find meaning in life. Furthermore, spiritual needs are the most fundamental requirement of the self. She offers the following descriptive characteristics of spirituality: Unfolding mystery, harmonious interconnectedness with self, others and a higher being, and inner strength or inner resources necessary for transcendence.

Spiritual Care

Nelms (1995) asserts that the origin of nursing is caring and that caring is its reason for being. Sourial (1997) differentiates between the technical services of care and the affective aspect of care and identifies an ethical imperative of nursing to care, incorporating technical and affective competence. She further identifies that caring is not the purview of nursing alone and therefore cannot be specific to nursing's role, however it does come within the purview of holism, which she identifies as a more comprehensive concept than caring.

Spiritual care is acknowledged in descriptions of nursing interventions, and although freely accepted, spiritual care, like spirituality, is not as easily described. During times of illness, pain, suffering and stress, people search for meaning, a spiritual quest that can lead to insight and healing, or fear and isolation (Fontaine, 2000; Travelbee, 1969; Carroll, 2001). Wright (1998) goes so far as to say that spiritual care is not only an integral aspect of nursing care, but to ignore spiritual care would be unethical on the part of the nurse. Ross (1994) reinforces that spiritual care is a nursing responsibility, not an optional extra, but adds that such care is hindered by a lack of a clear definition of spirituality and the absence of a conceptual framework from which to deliver such care. Reed (1992) adds that spirituality is foundational to nursing because it provides the basic characteristic of human-ness, and is essential to human well-being.

Quantitative studies of spirituality have been conducted largely with regard to religiosity. The concept of spirituality was studied using various Likert type scales and questionnaires. Richards (1991) studied 268 undergraduate students enrolled in general psychology courses at the University of Minnesota, who volunteered for the project. Using results of the Religious Orientation Scale, he divided the subjects into four groups: intrinsically religious, extrinsically religious, pro-religious, and anti-religious. Richards then used the Center for Epidemiology Studies Depression Scale, the Spiritual Well-being Scale and the Existential Well-Being Scale. Richards had hypothesized that non-religious students would exhibit more depression than religious students. Results did not bear this out. The implication is that spiritual dimensions are not limited to religiosity.

Giblin (1997) studied marital satisfaction with relation to marital spirituality. Subjects were 35 self-selected couples who belonged to marital support or prayer groups known to the author. Instruments used were all Likert style scales and included the Barrett-Lennard Relationship Inventory (RI), Spiritual Experience Index (SEI), Spiritual Well-being Scale (SWBS) and ENRICH, a multifaceted relationship functioning questionnaire. The author identified the subjects as predominantly Catholic, well educated, middle class and married for greater than 20 years, factors that would limit generalizability. Overall, results showed a significant correlation between ENRICH and SWBS and the mean score on RI and ENRICH were not significant. For husbands, spirituality was found to be directly related to marital relationships. For the wives, however, spirituality was separate from marital relationships. The author concluded that women are more oriented inward, introspective and oriented to developing and maintaining relationships.

In a 1987 study, Reed matched 300 adults into three groups: (1) non-terminally ill hospitalized, (2) terminally ill hospitalized, and (3) healthy non-hospitalized. Matching criteria included age, gender, years of education, and religious background. All subjects were from the same geographic area. All groups were administered the Spiritual Perspective Scale (SPS) in a structured interview setting. An Index of Well-Being was also administered to measure overall life satisfaction. Statistically significant differences were noted in SPS scores of the terminally ill hospitalized group compared to the non-terminally ill and healthy group combined; however no difference was found between non-terminally ill hospitalized and healthy non-hospitalized subjects. Findings supported the stated hypothesis that terminally ill hospitalized adults would indicate a greater spiritual perspective. The correlation between spiritual perspective and well being in the terminally ill group was weak, but significant. This relationship was not significant in the other two groups. It was also reported that a significantly larger number of terminally ill adults indicated a recent increase in spirituality than the other groups.

Touch is more than the procedure related contact of nurse and patient. It also includes that touch which conveys caring in the sense of 'being with' and connectedness, and as such, is an integral part of spiritual care. Mulaik, et al. (1991) studied patients' perceptions of touch in an exploratory study using a descriptive-comparative design. A convenience sample of 98 adults were administered the Patient Touch Questionnaire (PTQ), designed by the investigators, and the Interpersonal Behavior Survey (IBS). The PTQ had four subcategories: traditional touch, instrumental touch, optional touch and essential touch. Results indicated that patients see touch as indicative of caring and that touch by the nurses was important in care (93%). Some reported that touch also indicated control on the part of the nurse and should not be used often (59%). There was no indication on what type of touch (traditional, essential, optional or instrumental), or whether or not all touch was an indicator of control. The study indicated that more time was spent by nurses on instrumental touch such as giving medications, examining, etc. (frequency of about 6 events per day) than on optional touch, described as activities such as patting patients' hands or backrubs (frequency of less than one event per day).

PERCEPTION OF CARE

Latham (1996) investigated self-esteem as a predictor of perception of nursing care with 120 hospitalized adults using a combination of questionnaire completion and interview. The Krantz Health Opinion Survey (KHOS) was used to measure desire for control and Rosenberg's Self-Esteem Scale (SES) was used to estimate self-concept. Humanistic caring was measured by the Holistic Caring Inventory (HCI) resulting in four subscales of caring: physical, interpretive, spiritual, and sensitive, and the Supportive Nursing Behavior Checklist (SNBC). All were Likert scale questionnaires. Findings indicated that personal characteristics such as threat appraisal and coping techniques were important. In addition, younger patients visualized more coping alternatives and reported a higher valuing of nurse caring behaviors. Pain was also identified as a predictor of valuing nursing care. Overall, physical caring received a higher rating than spiritual caring. The author suggested that future research about personal characteristics of patients may lead to greater understanding of their perceptions of caring by nurses.

Holistic care involves not only patients themselves, but also family members. Eriksson (2001) studied relatives' of cancer patients perceptions of care received by their loved ones and developed a structured questionnaire for the study. A sample of 168 relatives from nine Finnish hospitals participated. Results indicated that the manner in which care was delivered was more important than the content of the care. The most important factor identified was professional skill, followed by safety, friendliness and professionalism. Relatives indicated they were more interested in information about the side effects of treatments and other aspects of care than they were in prognosis.

With regard to quality improvement based on patient perceptions of care and satisfaction, Drain (2001) sought to develop a survey instrument to evaluate patient experiences in order to improve quality of care. Findings indicated that perceptions of service affect perceptions of quality of care and that both satisfaction and quality of care perceptions should be evaluated to improve services to patients.

QUALITATIVE STUDIES

Spirituality, because of its lack of concreteness, does not lend itself well to quantitative measurement (Burkhart, 1989), which might be a reason for the limited amount of research in the area. Existential qualities of spirituality include but are not limited to joy, hope, peace, caring, courage, reverence, awe, and purpose in life. These concepts lend themselves more to qualitative measurement, in which subjectivity is valued in understanding the whole.

CARING BEHAVIORS

Halldorsdottir and Hamrin (1997) conducted a phenomenologic study of cancer patients that explored both caring and uncaring nursing behaviors as perceived by the patient. These researchers identified three caring behaviors: a) a companion in the "cancer trajectory", b) a mutual trust and caring, and c) a sense of well-being, solidarity, empowerment and healing (p. 122). They also identified three uncaring behaviors: a) perceived barrier to healing and well-being, b) mistrust and disconnection, and c) unease and discouragement.

In an effort to determine if patient's perceived caring needs were addressed in a new patient classification instrument, Fagerstrom, Eriksson, and Engberg (1999) interviewed 75 patients from Finland using a phenomenological-hermeneutical method. Seventeen caring needs were identified as a result. Twenty-three of the respondents expressed needs that encompassed the dimensions of body, mind and spirit as identified by the authors, however, physiologic needs were predominant in the needs identified. Caring needs included: to be seen holistically, comforted, well-being and security addressed, hope supported, guidance provided, welcomed, treated with dignity and to have devotional needs supported. The most consistent theme that emerged was that the nurse helped the patient to recover. Interestingly, perceived spiritual caring needs were not addressed in the classification system, while physical and psychological needs were. The authors suggested that the classification system be supplemented by a "caring perspective".

Nine women recovering from hip repair surgery were interviewed in a phenomenological study by Kralik, Koch and Wotton (1997) aimed at understanding what patients perceived as important about nursing care. Two major themes emerged: engagement and detachment. Engagement was supported by the minor themes of nurses approaching the patient in such a manner that conveyed that nothing was too much trouble in their care, consulting with the patient, smiling and using humor, having the qualities of being kind and compassionate, knowing what was needed without having to be asked, being available, friendly, warm, and using a gentle touch. The theme of detachment was supported by such perceived behaviors as "treating the patient as a number" (depersonalization), being too efficient or busy, conveying that the patient should "try harder" or encouraging to the extreme, not sharing information with the patient, even when asked, having "rough hands", and approaching the job of nursing as "just a job" or "just doing what they are told". From the patient's perspective, engagement was directly related to perceived quality of care.

Clark and Wheeler (1992) investigated the meaning of caring based on the experience of six staff nurses and concluded that caring incorporated four major categories: a) being supportive, b) communicating, c) caring ability, and d) pressure (meaning that the nurses believed that pressure and stress either in the workplace or in their personal lives impeded their ability to care). Nurses also indicated that the quality of care they perceived they gave was hindered by patients who "shut them off" (p. 1289).

In a 1999 Finnish qualitative study, Fredriksson synthesized research in nursing and caring utilizing hermeneutic analysis. Citing Nelms (1996), presence was described as both 'being there', which indicates attention by the nurse and 'being with', or an act of mutual giving and receiving. The latter making both giver and receiver more vulnerable in trusting and sharing. Touch was also interpreted to be either necessary to carry out a task, a form of nonverbal communication, or a protective strategy on the part of the nurse to reduce exposure to emotional pain. Listening was described as an active and deliberate attention to another, essential in developing a relationship. These three concepts, presence, touch and listening, were viewed as central to developing a caring conversation between nurse and patient.

Tumblin and Simkin (2001) examined pregnant women's perceptions of their expectations of the nurse's role in general during labor and delivery in an informal survey of women who had never had children. The women were surveyed in their third trimester, during a childbirth class. The survey asked participants to write responses to the question: "What do you think your nurse's role will be during labor and delivery?" (p. 53). Themes included physical comfort, emotional support, information and instructions, advocacy, and technical skills.

Radwin (2000) described eight attributes of quality nursing care: professionalism, knowledge, continuity as reflected by continued encounters, attentiveness, coordination of activities, partnership, individualization of the patient, rapport and caring. These attributes were described by cancer patients in a grounded theory study conducted in a Boston area medical center. Attributes of non-quality care were addressed in part by Hewison (1995) in an earlier observational study conducted in England. He concluded that most nurse/patient interactions were superficial, routine and talk-oriented. It was suggested that nurses exert a 'power over' relationship as indicated by language used in communication with their patients. This power attribute was perceived as a barrier to any meaningful communication. Larrabee and Bolden (2001) identified five themes in their qualitative descriptive study of 199 hospitalized adults. The themes were: providing for patient needs, treating the patient pleasantly, caring, being competent, and providing prompt care.

Appleton (1993) conducted a phenomenological hermeneutic study with 17 participants to identify nursing process as art. In this study, both nurses and patients provided descriptions of the nursing experience as art. Participants described nurses as being present when they focused on the patient as a whole person with the encounter as a temporal moment in the entirety of the lifespan. Patients indicated they wanted the nurse to be considerate and kind. The art of nursing was described by patients as very special when time was taken to care and the perception was that the nurses were giving their very best. From the nursing perspective, providing opportunities for patients to realize their potential was identified as part of the art of nursing. Themes included ways of being, being with, creating opportunities for fullness of being, transcendent togetherness and the context of caring.

Understanding the transactional nature of the basic care needs of patients was illustrated by a Danish study. Adamsen and Tewes (2000) conducted focus group interviews of 120 patients and 22 nurses in a Danish hospital addressing basic nursing care. Fully one third of the patient-identified problems with care were neither noted on the chart, nor known by the nurse caring for them. From the patient's perspective, basic care needs (e.g. pain management and nutritional needs) were being overlooked. Clearly nurses cannot meet needs of which they are unaware.

PATIENT EXPECTATIONS OF SPIRITUAL CARE

Two studies were identified that addressed specifically the spiritual aspect of care. Conco (1995) conducted a phenomenological study with 10 participants who identified themselves as Christian to determine what constituted spiritual care from the perspective of the patient. She identified three themes: enabling transcendence of the situation for a higher meaning, enabling hope and establishing connectedness. Conco concluded that connectedness was simply caring. Sellers (2001) interviewed six key and 12 general informants residing in the Midwest regarding their perceptions of spiritual nursing care. She identified five spiritual themes in this ethnonursing study: 1) Spirituality is a motivator in the search for meaning through connectedness; 2) Spirituality involves a lifelong search for meaning; 3) Spirituality is expressed and practiced uniquely; 4) The environment influences spirituality; and 5) Nurses can enhance spirituality by establishing a caring presence with both the patient and their family. According to Sellers, spiritual nursing care can be achieved by listening attentively to others' stories, individualizing care, approaching the patient with sensitivity and respect, and maintaining a good sense of humor.

From the perspective of client as the community, Chase-Ziolck and Gruca, 2000) studied religious congregations as a nontraditional site for nursing practice, with an emphasis on health promotion and spiritual care. The authors used naturalistic inquiry as a framework for their descriptive exploratory study of patients' perceptions of interacting with nurses in their congregations. Participants described ways they felt cared for by the nurse, to include 'being there' and 'being with'. Because the setting was in the community, emphasis was on interpersonal caring actions rather than technical caring actions. Several participants described the setting (their church) as supporting the feeling of tranquility, peace and care and illustrated the connection between faith and health.

Caring is identified as a universal culturally dependent phenomenon. With that premise, patient expectations of care were examined by Cortis (2000) in an ethno-linguistic study. Twenty male and eighteen female participants from a Pakistani community in the United Kingdom participated. There was a link between caring, culture and spirituality as demonstrated by the importance of relationships to self and others. The importance of developing the nurse-patient relationship in order for caring to be perceived was evident. As a whole, the perception was that nurses had limited observation, empathy, and communication skills, and that the "assessments they experienced had been mechanistic and ritualistic rather than the framework for developing a therapeutic relationship with them" (p. 59). The author concluded that more effective cultural assessment was needed to foster a therapeutic relationship.

SUMMARY

Quantitative studies regarding issues related to spiritual care and patient/family perceptions of care were limited mostly to Likert type questionnaire administration. Purpose in life studies revealed that commitment and psychological well-being were positively associated with purpose in life. Death anxiety, however was not. Quantitative studies of spirituality mainly measured elements of religiosity from the Judeo-Christian perspective. Findings revealed that spiritual dimensions were not limited to religiosity. Studies also support that terminally ill persons indicate a greater spiritual perspective. Touch was revealed to be important in care, however patients perceived instrumental touch (touching medications and machinery) more than personal touch (holding the hand). One study supported that self-esteem was a predictor of perception of nursing care and that pain was a predictor of perception of nursing care. Finally, studies support that the manner that care is delivered is more important to patients than the content of that care.

Qualitative studies examining the expectations of patients related to spiritual care were limited. For the most part, the literature addressed patient expectation themes of technical competence, caring, nursing as art, and quality of nursing. A meta-analysis gave more insight into care, but did not address specific spiritual themes. There was a significant amount of literature that addressed the ramifications of nursing care using the lens of the nursing shortage and managed care, all from the viewpoint of the nurse.

Caring behaviors were explored in several phenomenologic studies, identifying basic caring needs as: to be seen holistically, to be comforted, to have hope supported, to have guidance provided, to feel welcomed and to be treated with dignity. Additional caring behaviors identified included smiling, a gentle touch, for the nurse to be available, and to be treaded as a person, not a number. One study found nurses actual behaviors to be superficial and talk oriented. Only two studies addressed spiritual needs specifically. Themes that emerged included enabling hope, supporting connectedness to self, the nurse and to a higher power, and to facilitate search for meaning. Caring presence was seen as enhancing spiritual care.

Therefore, this literature review supports that spirituality is the essence of what it is to be human, and is central to health and the healing process. Nevertheless, it is difficult to define. Concepts associated with spirituality include hope, connection to self, others and a higher power, purpose or meaning in life, caring presence, religion, ritual, comfort, motivation, transcendence, well-being, values, beliefs, harmony, prayer or meditation, self-awareness, and even self-esteem. It is not evident whether or not these concepts are precursors of, or the result of spirituality.

Spirituality is often confused with, or a term used interchangeably with religion. Given that, spiritual needs are often referred by nurses to a chaplain or minister. No literature reviewed in this study addressed directly the spiritual needs of individuals who identify themselves as nonreligious or atheistic. Being a component of holism, spiritual care is within the purview of nursing. Indeed, it is an ethical responsibility of nursing.

A common thread in defining spirituality is that it involves a search for meaning or purpose in life, relationships with self, others and a higher being, and hope. The search for meaning or purpose in life can include any ideals or practices that contribute to a meaningful life. Meaning can only be ascribed by the individual. The role of the nurse in spiritual care is to understand the importance of spirituality to health and healing and to establish a trusting, caring relationship with the patient. It is not understood from the literature that patients would expect spiritual care from their nurse.

METHODOLOGY

Humanistic phenomenology is a framework for examining the lived experience of hospitalization and patients' expectations of care during that hospitalization. All participants were given an opportunity to reflect on their experience of hospitalization first by recounting their remembrances of their hospitalization by relating it in story form. Individual perceptions of hospitalization were very meaning-laden and as stories were elicited, the circumstances of hospitalization were expressed in words, gestures, tone and in a cadence unique to each participant.

Setting

The setting for this study was south-central United States. Two metropolitan statistical areas (MSA) located in bordering states were represented. Major economic influences for both MSAs included cattle, oil, and industries such as tire and tool manufacturing. Both MSAs serve a much wider rural population, and each are supported economically by separate military installations and small state universities. The larger MSA has a population of approximately 120,000 and the smaller, approximately 80,000.

Participants

Participants in this study were solicited via purposive sampling. Criterion sampling (soliciting interviews from any persons who meet the qualifications of the study and opportunistic sampling (following leads from participants and other informants) as described by Erlandson, Harris, Skipper, and Allen (1993) were used. The concepts of spirituality and perception of spiritual care are value laden and often used interchangeably with the concept of religion. Therefore, recruitment of participants evolved and, incorporating the strategy of maximum variation (Miles and Huberman, 1994), resulted in the solicitation of both self-identified religious and non-religious participants. Participants were interviewed until redundancy, which was indicated after nine interviews. In order to assure that no new substantive information would result from interview, two additional interviews were conducted. The quality of the content of the interviews indicated redundancy. Therefore, a total of 11 interviews were conducted. Data collection was conducted between May 2002 and January 2003.

Data Generation Strategies

All potential participants approached by the researcher consented to participate in the study. Participants were told that study participation would involve an interview lasting approximately one to two hours. All interviews were completed in about a one-hour time frame. The range of interview times was 30 minutes to 1 hours and 20 minutes. In order to elicit an unbiased sense of participants' expectations of nurses, the concept of spirituality was not mentioned as a focus of the study during participant recruitment with two exceptions. Some aspects of spirituality, such as building relationships, may not be recognized as such my the participants. It was important to get the flavor of the lived experience, which may have included aspects of spirituality, prior to introducing it as a topic and risking leading participants into telling the researcher what she wanted to hear. One participant was known to be atheistic. In order to assure that he was not "blindsided" by the interview questions regarding spirituality, he was told during recruitment that spirituality was an aspect of holistic nursing care and was a focus of the study. One participant knew through personal conversation, prior to recruitment, that the focus of the study was spirituality and requested to be included in the study. At the end of the interview, participants were told that one of the purposes of the research was to learn patients' expectations regarding spiritual care (as defined by holistic nursing standards of practice) from nurses. A written summary of the findings was available upon request to participants after compilation and analysis of the data. No participants indicated they wanted a summary of the findings.

Interviews were scheduled after either telephone or direct communication with potential participants. Informed consent was obtained at the time of the scheduled interview and a pseudonym of the participant's choosing was identified. Participants were asked, first to relate a story about a specific nurse or an experience with nursing care while they were hospitalized. Based on what the participant related, follow-up questions were asked in order to address the following basic questions:

1. What did you expect from your nurse when you were hospitalized?
2. How do you define or describe good nursing care?

3. Did you expect spiritual care from a nurse?
4. How do you define or describe spiritual nursing care?

Again, depending on the responses, nursing behaviors considered by nurses to embody the spiritual dimension of holistic practice would be offered, such as, "The spiritual component of care includes developing a trusting relationship with your nurse so that those things that give meaning to your life, such as art, music, meditation, relationships, or faith are acknowledged, supported and facilitated." I provided this definition if participants defined spiritual care only in terms of religious practice in order to elicit deeper description or discussion of the term "spiritual" or "spirituality". Therefore, I provided my definition in five of the eleven interviews.

Interviews were conducted at a time convenient to the participants, at a place of their choosing. Eight participants chose to be interviewed in my office. The office door was closed and distractions were minimal. Three participants were interviewed in their own business offices per their request. All interviews were audiotaped with permission. Audiotapes were used in this study to insure the accuracy of interview date as well as to record the exact words, tones, and emphasis conveyed by the participants. The reasons for this were twofold. First, meaning is conveyed by more than just words alone. Pauses, sighs, time for reflection, tone, choice of words, and voice modulation are also important in gleaning the full meaning of the words. Second, I could focus attention on being present with the participant and his/her interview rather than being distracted by constant note-taking. This attention during the interview would help to establish a trusting relationship. Audiotapes were only available to the participant and the principal investigator. While the proposed interview content had been piloted in interviews already conducted and found to elicit responses related to the topic, I remained flexible and use further clarifying questions as needed in each specific situation.

Two participants became tearfully emotional during the interview process. These two participants were given the option of terminating the interview or the audiotaping, and both elected to continue with the audiotaped interview process. All participants were told that they could contact me at any time after the interview for questions or additional comments. No participants contacted me for additional questions or comments. Participants did ask some questions during the course of the interview itself. In order to not interrupt the flow of the participant's stories, demographic data that were not made apparent during the course of the interview were collected at the end of the interview process. Demographic data included age, gender, race/ethnicity, marital status, religious preference, number and ages of children, diagnosis for which hospitalized, number of hospitalizations, level of education, occupation, and age at the time of hospitalization.

Interviews began with having each participant tell a story about being hospitalized. This strategy was appropriate. First, rich data were obtained. Second, participants seemed to become more at ease as they progressed in the telling of their story. Several participants were very concerned about the details such as dates, times, and names of their physician – the facts of their hospitalization – as they began their narratives. As they became immersed in the storytelling, I noticed that the event itself took on more importance. The narratives dictated follow-up questions.

Plan for Data Analysis

Audiotapes were made of each interview and transcribed verbatim. The analysis method described by Giorgi (1970) fit well with the data obtained and my own personal thought processes. Data were then analyzed using the phenomenologic method described by the psychologist Giorgi to identify patterns and themes. This method is based on reflection, an ordered, repetitive examination of the data to derive implications and meaning. Procedurally, the steps of the Giorgi method are:

1. Interview the participants.
2. Read the description (verbatim transcription) to get a sense of the whole.
3. Re-read and reflect on the description several times and identify individual units (patterns and themes).
4. Eliminate redundancies in the patterns and themes, clarifying each by relating them to each other and to the whole.
5. Continue to reflect on the patterns and themes, transforming meaning from concrete language into the language or concepts of the science (nursing literature).
6. Integrate and synthesize meaning into descriptive structure communicated to others.

I transcribed all interviews. After transcription, I read through each transcribed interview while listening to the audiotape until I was sure of accuracy of the transcription and had reflected on the meaning of the interview. Any additional nuances of tone, inflection and pause in narrative were noted in this process. An interview summary was written for each interview, to include exemplars of any themes or patterns noted.

Steps to Insure Methodological Rigor

Credibility was established by this investigator's 18 years of nursing experience and having prolonged engagement with the participants. Each interview lasted between 30 minutes and one hour 20 minutes. In addition, member checks were accomplished by requesting elaboration or clarifying concepts with each participant during the course of their interview. After reflecting on the interviews and rereading transcriptions, no questions arose that required follow-up interviews. No participant contacted me after the interview to add any comment or clarification. A nurse colleague, experienced in phenomenological methodology was asked to review the transcribed interviews (with participant aliases) and provide feedback regarding her impression of the interviews and to discuss emergent themes and patterns. This peer debriefing was ongoing throughout the data analysis process.

Transferability was addressed by eliciting rich description and providing thick description of the interviews. Any pertinent noises, sights, facial expressions, gestures and tones were included in field notes. Sampling was purposive to insure maximum variability of the phenomena of perceptions of nursing care during hospitalization.

Dependability and confirmability of the data were addressed by an audit trail to include audiotapes, transcriptions of the interviews, field notes of the investigator, notes of the peer debriefer, and interview summaries of each interview. I kept notes on the interview transcript and added to those notes each time I reread the transcripts as warranted. These notes addressed general impressions of the interviews, the settings, collaborative data, and historical data, which might impact the tone of the interview. For example, one participant consented to be interviewed and subsequently was diagnosed with a terminal illness. Concerned that the interview timing would not be in this person's best interest, I offered this participant the option of not being interviewed. She declined, stating that she really wanted to talk about her hospitalization. I believe the interview process was cathartic for this individual.

A methodological decision was made, for ethical reasons, to inform one prospective participant that spirituality and spiritual care would be discussed when soliciting his participation. Methodologically, this topic was not going to be addressed prior to the interview to attempt to avoid having participants "tell the researcher what she wants to hear". This participant was known to be atheistic, and I believed that he might feel entrapped without this information up front. He chose to participate and even brought Internet sites and literature to the interview to, as he stated, help me to understand his belief system.

Protection of Human Participants

None of the participants voiced any concern for loss of confidentiality, however, the principal investigator was the only individual with access to the identity of the participants. Pseudonyms (aliases) were self-assigned by the participants. Two participants became tearful during the course of their interviews, but both elected to continue the interviews. One participant referred to family members by name during the course of their interview and requested that the family member's name not be used. The family member's name was not used. No participant voiced any concern about being audiotaped.

DEMOGRAPHIC DATA

A total of seven women and four men participated in the study. The age range of participants was 36 to 59 years. All participants self-identified as Caucasian. All participants graduated from high school. Three participants had 2 to 3 years of college, five had baccalaureate degrees, one had a masters degree and two participants possessed doctoral degrees. Three participants self-identified as secretaries, one as a homemaker, one as a teacher, two as students, one as a broadcast engineer, two as university professors, and one as a retired police officer. Ten of the participants were married and one was in a committed relationship. Ten reported having 1 to 3 children while two reported having no children. The range of number of hospitalizations (requiring at least one overnight stay) of the participants was 1 to 13 times. Religious preference of the participants included Protestant (two Baptist, one Methodist, one Disciple of Christ, one Presbyterian, one Episcopalian, and one no-preference), Catholic (one), Agnostic (two), and Atheist (one).

FINDINGS

The experience of hospitalization evoked strong feelings on the part of the participants, both positive and negative. The nature of the disease process and the number of times hospitalized varied with the participants, but it was clear that each experienced a sense of vulnerability, exacerbated by uncertainty that contributed to the event of their hospitalization being a very significant life event. Although each related experience was unique, there were some commonalities among participants in the experience of hospitalization and with the nurses who provided their care. Four major themes emerged in data analysis (Davis, 2005):

1.   Definitions of "good" and "bad" nursing care
2.   Expectations of surveillance and competence
3.   Spiritual care expectations and definitions
4.   Time and the nursing shortage

The focus of this paper will be spiritual care expectations and definitions. While all participants were able to define what they believed to be spiritual care and spirituality, nine of the 11 participants did not expect spiritual care from their nurses. In fact, one adamantly did not want it. Spiritual care was chiefly defined in terms of religious affiliation or religious practices or rituals such as prayer. Nurse referral to a chaplain or minister was, in general, thought to be the extent of nursing involvement in spiritual care. When provided with my definition of spiritual care, developing a trusting relationship with the nurse so that those things that give meaning to life such as art, music, meditation, relationships, or faith are acknowledged, supported and facilitated, participants generally agreed that spiritual care, thus defined, would be good for the nurse to do, but did not expect it. Shorter lengths of hospital stay, that preclude developing a relationship with the nurse, and workload of nurses were offered as rationales for not expecting spiritual nursing care.

Robbi had no expectations of spiritual care, but stated she would like to experience it, "I find it very comforting when I realize that the nurse and I have that connection." Lena also had no real expectations, but she articulated, "I usually think of it in terms as being requested by the patient. It sort of takes a request by the patient in a formal sense, someone to pray with or read literature with or whatever."

George defined spiritual care as something to be referred to the minister and would not expect spiritual interaction from nurses, citing lack of time on the part of the nurse. Even so, he gave the impression that nurses are not expected to attend to every wish of the patient, but to their needs, and spiritual care was not considered to be a need in the hospital setting.

> [Nurses are] extremely busy. I think most patients realize that. It's sort of like you're not expecting you know, a body servant or anything, or there as a personal kind of a counselor. You're mostly there as an individual patient that just has to wait their turn. You don't really look on it as the be all and end all. You don't see them really all that often. If you call on them they arrive, or something that has to be done procedurally they'll be there, but other than that, you hardly ever see them. They don't come in and say 'hi, how are you feeling' or generally chit chat for a little while... Well, I'm sure that if they had time, it would be nice.

Carol became tearful and was given the option of terminating the interview when spirituality was introduced as a topic. She was recently diagnosed with a terminal illness and had been in and out of the hospital for testing and pain management several times over the weeks preceding the interview. She began discussing the fact that she was not a deeply religious person. Although raised in a religious household, Carol began to question the religion she grew up with when she stated college and "reading more", to include reading about evolution. She went on to describe her feelings regarding religion and a higher being, stating that it just "didn't add up", referring to creation theory and the presence of a higher being. When asked to describe spiritual nursing care she described emotional comforting, a 'being with' on the part of the nurse. However, her conception of spirituality was mainly religion and religious practices, and the role of the nurse was limited to referral if indicated to a minister.

> I would think it would be a nurse coming in and telling me that 'you're going to get through this', possibly offering to get a minister in if I wanted one or something like that. I don't look on it as somebody taking my hand and saying a prayer with me. I don't look on it as that. I think if you want spiritual guidance or you want spiritual help that a nurse is going to know how to get it for you.

After hearing my definition of spiritual care, Carol was thoughtful, and agreed that all individuals have something that is important, that gives meaning, to them. She added that it is important to know someone, to develop a trusting relationship with the nurse, for some issues related spiritual care, such as things that give meaning to life, to be shared with another. When a more personal relationship develops with the nurse, she believed that this more personal information was shared because the patient feels more comfortable.

> Those things come out. Like you might say music relaxes me. You would you expect the nurse to pick up on that and offer to bring in a radio or something. That, to me would be providing spiritual care to you... Some people are annoyed by music. Every person has something that is extremely important, to me.

Diane did not expect spiritual care from her nurse, but when asked what it was, she could clearly describe it. Diane saw spiritual care as multidimential. Elements of caring presence, 'being with', what she terms "people skills", such as being gentle, unhurried, developing a relationship, were included in her definition of spiritual care. She added that nurses should not detract from the healing environment of the hospital. Basically, if the nurse can't help, at least he/she should not be harmful, and this is included in the spiritual care of the patient.

> ...Like don't rush out of the room. Skills, actual people skills that could be taught that, and one is gentle tone of voice, touch gently. Maybe they don't give a hoot about you, but, you're not worse for their coming in the room. You know, you are not worse for connecting with them. They [nurses] say, 'do you want anything' and you are trying to answer and then before you know it... they're gone. [Laughs] Actually, now that you say it, connectedness is exactly what it takes. An actual concern, you know. I think you can draw pain away from people or do things for people. It's kind of a Christian based belief -that we can lift our burdens kind of thing. It's to form some kind of bond, [along] with that, empathy and sincerity. That you involve yourself enough to lift some of the burden off the patient. If someone can take you out of yourself for a moment. So, there you go.
> Being recognized as an individual was considered to be part of spiritual care.

Carol also related that being made to "feel human" was important to spiritual care and was important to her. She indicated that she was comforted when the nurse wanted to help her, even if she was capable of caring for herself, because she saw that as acknowledging her, that she was seen as having worth as a human being.

Just make you feel human. ...I appreciate that more than anything. You know, I'm not a problem patient. I'd just as soon do something myself than to ring a buzzer and have someone do it for me. And, I like to be acknowledged that way, you know, like, 'Mrs. ____ why didn't you call me to do that'. Oh, I'm fine. I can do it. 'Well next time call me.' [laughs] You know ... most of the nurses are like that.

Mary also found it helpful to be recognized as an individual. She recounted that nurses who cared for her when she was hospitalized for pneumonia treated her as a "whole person", which greatly enhanced the healing environment. This sense of acknowledgement as a human being was accomplished by nurses taking time to form a personal relationship with her. Mary's perception was that the nurses were fully present with her in their interactions.

...and the nurses who took care of me here at [hospital] really made me feel like they cared about me as a whole person. There was a man nurse and a number of women nurses and, I really got the impression that they didn't think of me as the lungs in room 406, that they thought of me as this real person, who's sick and we're going to treat the whole person and try to get better. They would take the time to visit with me and I knew they had all the people they had to see and all the meds they had to get out and this enormous amount of work to deal with, and they would spend a few minutes to see how I was doing as a person in addition to dealing with the pneumonia. But they really made me feel like they cared about me as a whole person.

Mary further clarified that the sense of being treated as a whole person was enhanced by the fact that the nurses talked to her. In addition to the verbal communication, demeanor and body language contributed to the overall sense of being cared for by nursing staff.

Some of it was the talking itself. Some of it was the nonverbal communication, the looks on their faces, the, probably open body language although I couldn't tell you that. So, I'm going to say probably it was the body language thing, facial features and open body language. But I really did feel like they cared about me more than just the lungs in 608.

David, self identified as atheistic, was told that spiritual care, as an element of holistic care would be included in the interview when he was recruited in an effort to ensure that David did not feel entrapped as the interview progressed. As a result, although he consented to the interview,

David conducted the majority of his interview in a defensive mode, leaning forward in his chair with hand on his knees and he seemed to have prepared some comments prior to arriving at the interview. In fact, he brought an article printed from an Internet site, written by a physician, supportive of atheistic beliefs. As the interview progressed, he seemed to become more at ease, leaning back in his chair and pausing more between responses. At the conclusion of the interview, he continued to converse about atheism and spirituality. He strongly associated the word "spiritual" with religious beliefs, which he was ardently opposed to, and therefore was opposed to the word. He believed that the term "meaningful" was more helpful than "spiritual" for nurses to use in their definition of holistic care, and that there were things that gave meaning to life, such as music. He did not, however, expect the nurse to be concerned with what he found meaningful in life, including developing any personal kind of relationship with his nurse. He stated that providing comfort was appropriate but believed that nurses should operate under the axiom of "doing no harm", to include care that the patient might "need" as opposed to "want", the implication being that providing the patient with what they want might be doing harm. David also stated that he did not have the expectation that the nurse be able to intuit what the patient might want. If the patient wants something, according to David, he or she must ask for it.

> I think there are great limits to that [spiritual care] and great dangers that the nurse has to be aware of. You know.... should a nurse pray with a patient if the patient is praying for the strength not to get a blood transfusion and they don't get the blood transfusion? If they might die—should the nurse aid and abet that wish to make the patient feel more comfortable with that? How does that conflict with the Hippocratic oath? And I think her duty to medicine and her duty to science and her duty to patient care should always supercede what the patient wants if there is a potential conflict.

Although most participants identified religious aspects of spirituality such as prayer and developing a relationship to a higher being, definitions of spiritual care included referral to nature, connectedness to self and others, and music. Robbi stated that the nurse conveys the spiritual side of care by her actions. In addition, she stated that spirituality includes getting to know someone and the "little things like family or pets that you're interested in." She also mentioned nature as spiritual, and important to her. She implied that nature was one of those "little things" which could be shared in building a relationship with her nurse.

...don't you just love it when the trees leaf out? There are some questions that, on the surface, sound very unimportant, but I think they convey a lot about a person and how they connect with the earth and, you know, as a part of each of us.

Lena spoke of spirituality having a formal and an informal component. She described her early experience with what she termed a fundamentalist religion with very strict and judgmental practices. She had since rejected those fundamentalist beliefs. Her life choices were not congruent with the religious practices of her childhood and of her family. She was divorced and entered into a lesbian relationship. These life choices continued to create angst in that her family members condemned her lifestyle choices based on their religious beliefs. Clearly, Lena was a spiritual person, but maintained no religious affiliation. Lena reflected that spirituality had a formal or religious component as well as an informal component that included sympathy, empathy and reassurance.

I think the way I define spiritual for myself personally is a much more informal thing. And its much more about that sensitivity and providing someone empathy or reassurance. Or in cases you can't really reassure as much, because you've lost something you're not going to get back, but ... just offer to listen, and sympathy are much more important than that formal spiritual advisor or leader. I think if I was hospitalized today, I would still be the same way, I wouldn't necessarily be looking for anyone to come and pray with me or read the Bible to me but I would feel better just having someone to talk to for a little bit. Or to listen to me, or to let me cry, you know... You know that informal [spirituality] I think is more important for me personally, because I think you spiritually minister to someone through those [listening and offering sympathy and reassurance]. And it's completely, its nondenominational, or not church affiliated in any way. And it wouldn't matter to me if the nurse were Christian, Jewish, Hindu, Islamic. I mean, that part would not be important to me. These are their own personal beliefs. But you know I come from a very conservative fundamentalist Christian background and in my life I have found that [pause] that whole viewpoint as - people from that kind of background tend to convert people, think that they can be saved, comfort people, aren't very comforting really at all and in fact are really offensive to me, you know. You know, all those things I have heard growing up over and over again. And that would upset me if I had a nurse come in and say those kinds of things to me. I would have a real problem with that.

Mart offered more insight into differences in religious and spiritual beliefs and indicated that, if the nurse held a different belief, spiritual care may be detrimental to the patient. She brought up a very salient point. She reinforced the point that all religious practices are not the same, even within the same religious heritage. Mary self-identified as Episcopalian. She strongly believed that denominational religious beliefs are not necessarily the same. She also strongly believed in the power of prayer and was concerned when anyone offered to pray for her. Because of the differences in beliefs, it was possible that, however well-meaning, the proffered prayer may be in contradiction with her beliefs. She defined spirituality as "a connection between myself and a higher power", but was clear that there was no expectation of spiritual care from her nurse, in fact, it would not be welcome.

> ... and I don't expect my nurses to do anything related [to spirituality]. In fact...I'm Episcopalian. And, people of other denominations say they're praying for me, it often annoys me because their belief systems are so very different from mine, so no I really don't expect spiritual care from the nurse.

Because Mary valued being treated as a whole person, I attempted to further clarify if spirituality was included in her definition of holism. When asked about her definition of holism from an education standpoint, she responded.

> That we educate not just the mind, ah, intellectually, but we are concerned with what we call the whole child. We're concerned with social relationships that the kids, about how he deals with his family, we're concerned that his physical needs be met - his nutrition, is he well. So we're concerned, but we draw a very sharp line between spiritual and non-spiritual kinds of concerns because of, if we step on the line, and I know some horror stories of... one that comes to mind right now is a little first grader whose dog died, and was crying and one of his teachers- The child said, 'my dog died, will he go to heaven?' and she said no, honey, I'm sorry, but dogs don't go to heaven. And, ah, of course this kid was traumatized. So, we draw a real hard line that we don't involve ourselves in anything spiritual. Physical self is cared for and the social self is cared for and certainly the intellectual self is cared for.

Given her definition of holism, Mary was asked if she expected that from her nurse. She responded in the affirmative, "Yeah, I expect that from my nurse. I expect her to be concerned and to be sure: Do I have any family? Am I getting um, cards coming? And are people coming to visit me?"

Lee referred to relationships in his definition of spiritual nursing care. Important relationships for him included those of family. Also important to him was developing a relationship with his nurse. He identified caring as the key component of spiritual nursing care. He also viewed coaching, encouraging and exhibiting genuine concern as key to spiritual care.

> ...my family being there for some of my surgeries, you know, I really want them to know what's going on, Let em know 'he's doing fine'. [pause] As far as the music...that doesn't play a part so much. Bottom line is caring. To me that's spiritual. Caring for your patient, caring for your [the patient's] parents, or your family that are asking questions also...You know, you're flat on your back and pretty helpless. Having somebody there who's going to take care of you. Every factor. Whether it's you know, a sponge bath, or taking you to the restroom, or you know, waiting for you to come out, you know, wheeling you here and there if you have to. Pushing. That's a big thing too. Pushing me to get up and get around... Coaching. Coaching me a little bit. And ah, wanting to see you get better, and wanting to see you leave. Not to get rid of you, but you know that you've made it through it and you're going to be fine... I think you have to have kind of a bond, a rapport. If you get off on a bad foot, you may not get someone. You know, pain in the butt, you're not going to get anything. It goes with personality also. You know, personality of the patient and the nurse.

He added that he did expect spiritual care, developing a bond and coaching, from his nurse, but stated, "I think that it makes the recovery time and the hospital stay a lot nicer."

Harold defined spirituality as "...kind of leans toward the religious aspect of things. But, I am not one who needs this." However, although he did not need or expect spiritual nursing care, he acknowledged that some patients do have religious needs when in the hospital and the nurse should have the skill to intuit such need.

> This is a case of a nurse needs to learn, I think, to be able to read a person and read something along those lines...To kinda bring the obvious out in the open. Give you a light you've never seen before. Give you an idea.... where you can help yourself. They can help you bring this out... Of course if they know how. And it should be taught.

Debbie, a nursing educator, did not expect spiritual nursing care. She defined spirituality more in terms of her own religious beliefs, to include prayer. She agreed with my definition of spiritual nursing care, however, and went on to describe an incident in which she allowed family members to visit a patient outside of visiting hours because she knew it was important and a comfort to her Hispanic patient. She added that, with caring, you are "sensitive to what that patient needs for support. And then you do as much as you can to give that support."

Diane saw religion as different from spirituality. This distinction was revealed at the end of the interview when gathering demographic data. When asked if she had a religious preference, she replied that religion and spirituality were two different things. She defined religion as an "organized, group of same faithed believers who gather and share to express worship." She envisioned spirituality as,

> Well spirituality to me is connectedness to the whole, with God. First with God, and then, through that, is connectedness with everything, and that has nothing to do with religion. Although, I can see where you get there through religion, or that's a good way to teach about, faith, or God or the Bible, Talmud, but spirituality to me is that communication with God, connectedness with God or with [something] larger than yourself. That there is, you know, life or being beyond your limits. Like we're all cells in an organism. The organism is God, maybe. When I hear, 'we are of God', I believe that. I feel a part of something, whether it's through my thoughts or deeds or actions, I feel like it affects everything around me almost. What we do matters. I mean, I don't go around, I'm not a peace nut or anything, and I have bad days, but I think it affects other people and I don't think its right to do those things. And the reason I think we're connected is because I don't have a way of not believing in God. I can't. We're all part of something bigger. We're all blades of grass. Mostly we're connected because of the world. We live on this planet together. If there are lots of possibilities there will be wars here or there or there are lots of possibilities there will be shooting, I just can't take the stress of the hostility and people are mean and the government doesn't care, and the first person they see on the subways spits on them. I understand that. I'm a part of that, so I have to care about it. Even evolution just blows my mind. Music is almost a direct line to spirituality. It's a healing sort of thing. That's another thing. Some people heal better through some visual or auditory stimuli, at least for me... That's another thing, taking a walk it the morning. And music, almost puts you in a meditative state. The way to concentrate is to get out of your normal way of thinking and it's very external. When you walk, your senses, all that input from nature can overwhelm. Just to breath. But music, you hear as well as play. Right away, playing music can put me in a better state- calm. And if I'm not in a place to play music, then listening, but playing is a different thing.

Listening's fine, but it's not the same. Falling into it. Music and art, why would you do that if you didn't have hope or being compelled to make something beautiful almost, or to create. What's the point of that if [voice trails off]. There's something it does."

David, an atheist, objected to the term "spiritual" because of the religious connotations, but did see himself as a whole being, not distinguishing between mind, body and personality. He viewed spirituality as a label that had no meaning to him.

I don't know what spirit means and I don't believe in the duality of body and mind. My brain is my mind. There is no such thing as of mind and of body. Without the body there is no mind so I don't see the point in splitting the two... I'm a very analytical, laid back kind of person, and I think labels like that would probably best describe my personality most of the time. Everybody has down or off days in terms of characteristics, but I can display the other ones at times, but those [analytic and laid back personality] are probably my dominant ones.

When I related the definition of spirituality I had developed, he replied that the term "meaningful" as opposed to "spiritual" was a good label:

Well then I would term meaningful as a good label there, and philosophical probably a better label as well, because the word spiritual has way too much other baggage attached to it that I don't buy into. So,... if nurses are to provide fulfillment in patient's philosophical realm and help make their experience as being meaningful to them then, if that assertion is true then I think those are better labels to use. But if that is, if my definition is what you mean by spiritual then feel free to use it [the term spiritual] as linguistic shorthand [basically giving permission to use the term, spiritual] as long as we both understand what we are talking about."

Toward the end of the interview, when responding to demographic data, David identified religious preference as "atheist' and seemed to be watching me carefully to gauge my reaction to this. We both stood and moved toward the door. At this point, David seemed to be less guarded and asked, good-humoredly, if there was anything else he could "spout off" about. It was as if he could relax now that the formal part of the interview was over. He suggested that using the word "mood" instead of "spirit" would be more appropriate.

I still don't like the term spiritual, but I'm very uh, you know, who wouldn't be spiritual if it's defined the way you are defining it... How's your mood. That's a way of assessing spirit. Feeding the spirit—keeping the mood stable and healthy. If you're somebody who's questioning some very deeply held beliefs - that can be a very painful disturbing process. Does that mean its bad? Should a nurse try to alleviate that, or should she try to encourage you, or should she just stay out of it and stick to giving meds to make you feel better physically, and respect the boundaries of your personal conscious and thinking and decisions on matters like that?

DISCUSSION

Humanistic nursing is predicated on the assumption that, while each person is unique, and each patient will respond uniquely to care, however, humans are more alike than different and value is also placed on that common humanness (Patterson and Zderad, 1985). While Benner (1985) and Rogers (1972) clearly indicate that nurses cannot understand health and illness by studying only the mind and body, but by studying the whole in context, it is believed that understanding the experience of the spiritual dimension of care will enhance the integrality of holistic care. Because of the existential nature of humanistic nursing, what nurses do should be perceived by patients in their care (Patterson and Zderad, 1985). Discussion will be organized around the research questions of this study.

1. Are the Explicit and Implicit Actions of Nurses to Address Body, Mind and Spirit Recognized by their Patients?

Participants in this study were able to discern actions by nurses, both implicit and explicit, which addressed holistic care as well as implicit and explicit actions by nurses, which detracted from holistic care. Actions addressing physical care (the body) were readily discernable and described. Actions which addressed mind and spirit were also readily discernable and described, but not necessarily using the terminology of mind and spirit. In stories of hospitalization in general, and when asked to relate a story of good nursing care, patients were able to distinguish qualities of good nursing care and bad nursing care. Good nursing care included descriptions of experiences congruent with holistic nursing care, to include spirituality. Participants described being made to feel special or being treated as a human being, and good nurses as being kind, caring, and willing to share themselves. Of note, the stories of both good and bad nursing care were very vivid and detailed, even though some of the instances occurred over 30 years ago. Bad nursing care, as described by the participants, was the antithesis of good nursing care, and included behaviors suggesting lack of kindness and lack of caring, such as talking about a patient in a derogatory manner in the hall, not meeting basic care needs, addressing the patient with a lack of respect, and not seeing the patient as an individual. Good and bad nursing care seemed to have such an impact on the participants that incidents of good and bad nursing care were easily and vividly recalled. As Cathy, who recalled neither good nor bad nursing care from her hospitalization pointed out, " You know, you remember things like that, and I have no negative memories".

Good nursing care was described very clearly and articulately. Data were similar to those reported by Sellers (2001) in her study of Christian patients' perceptions of spiritual nursing care. Participants in that study were also able to describe effective and ineffective nursing care. Effective care reflected elements such as caring presence, compassion, active listening, respect, and a sense of humor. Sellers reported ineffective care as participants perceiving they were not being seen as a person; that nurses were insensitive or focused on procedures. Body, mind and spirit were addressed in the concept of presence as described by Benner (1985), to include both 'being there' and 'being with', and were described by patients in their narratives about good nursing care. Benner, in her description of expert nursing care found that the personhood and dignity of the patient were recognized by the expert nurse and the resultant actions of the nurse were perceived by the patient. Physical presence, 'being there', involves touching, assessing, doing, hearing and represents the routine level of physical nursing care, whereas psychological or therapeutic presence, 'being with', involves the therapeutic use of self, to include both verbal and nonverbal communication, with the intention of establishing a meaningful connection with the patient (Taylor, 2002; Watson, 1999).

Participants in this study had an expectation of competence of their nurses which was addressed in the physical presence, 'being there', of the nurse. These participants expressed an expectation of nursing knowledge and skill, correct, prompt attention to physical needs, administering medications in a timely manner, and assessing and attending to pain. Sourial (1997) proposed that physical care was perceived as more important to patients than psychosocial or existential care, and that nurses may take physical care for granted, in that physical care was seen as an imperative, whereas psychosocial or existential care was only provided if there was time. Eriksson (2001) likewise identified professional skill as important to perception of care. Latham (1996) reported that, overall, physical care was of more value to patients than spiritual care. This was certainly reflected in the stories and expectations verbalized by participants in this study. Physical care was a universal expectation and was universally valued by the participants in this study. Participants expected physical care more than they expected spiritual care. Spiritual care was greatly valued, but not expected.

Brush and Daly (2000) use the terms 'being here' and 'being there', and assert that presence is essential in spiritual caregiving. Although not specifically identified as elements of spirituality, study participants stressed that being seen as an individual, as a human being, was important. 'Being there' was a cardinal element in participants' descriptions of good nursing care and reflected 'being there' as described by Brush and Daly or the more common term in the literature, 'being with' (Benner, 1985; Burkhardt and Nagai-Jacobson, 2002; Chase-Ziolck et al, 2000; Nelms, 1996; Taylor, 2002; and Watson, 1999). Arthur Frank (1991), a trained sociologist, was profoundly affected by his own experience with illness and wrote of this experience with illness and hospitalization. He stressed that care only begins when differences (individualities) are recognized. Participants in the current study described good nursing care as being seen as individuals, as a human being. Caring was perceived as more than attending to physical needs in a technically competent manner only if the participants were seen as individuals. These data indicate that while the commonality of being human gives value, being seen as an individual allows persons/humans to feel valued; and the feeling of value is predicated by being cared for as an individual with a disease or health condition, not treated as a disease or health condition of a human. Most poignantly, "The common diagnostic categories into which medicine places its patients are relevant to disease, not to illness. They are useful for treatment, but they only get in the way of care (Frank, 1991, p. 45)".

Sharing of self by the nurse was a recurrent concept in the data. It was described as an integral part of being accepted as an individual by the nurse and of developing a trusting relationship. This humanistic holistic perspective, to include compassion, was also reflected as being considerate, kind and pleasant by participants. These characteristics were also described by Appleton (1993) as desires of patients. More than performing tasks, presence requires an openness on the part of the nurse to 'being with' a patient (Burkhardt and Nagai-Jacobson, 2002), and that openness reveals both the being of the nurse and the being of others, to include the patient (Nelms, 1996).

Appleton (1993) conceptualized the 'other' aspect of presence - that of patient presence, and the patient's way of being there as someone needing care and feeling vulnerable during hospitalization. The response of the nurse to the patient's presence would then result in comfort and reduced vulnerability. The participants' desires for touch, both touch needed for physical care, and comforting touch, are explicit in the concept of caring presence. Touch is identified in the theoretical literature as an element of presence (Burkhardt and Nagai-Jacobson, 2002; Swanson, 1999; Watson, 1999) and in research literature as indicative of caring (Fredriksson, 1999; Mulaik et al, 1991). Participants in the current study described being vulnerable and of being comforted in their descriptions of good nursing care. Data suggested a lack of comfort and a continued sense of vulnerability in stories of bad nursing care. I conclude that the hallmark of the conceptualization of good nursing care seemed to focus on existential spiritual care activities that the nurse performed that helped to reduce those feelings of vulnerability, specifically, not only seeing patients as human beings, but treating patients with kindness, gentleness and comforting touch. The mutuality of presence, both recognizing patients' presence as described by Appleton and offering nursing presence, is consistent with the existential nature of humanistic nursing and my assumption that nursing is holistic. Recognizing the presence of the patient and responding with caring presence, to include interventions of comforting touch, kindness, gentleness, and recognizing individuality are not expectations of patients when hospitalized, but are certainly recognized and appreciated as elements of good nursing care.

Adamsen and Tewes (2000) found a discrepancy in patient perception of the care they received and the care perceived as being giving by nursing staff. Perceptions of pain, sleep and rest, and problems that impact quality of life, although generally recognized by nursing staff, were underestimated by nursing staff according to patient perceptions. There was some evidence that this perception of care also occurred in the narratives provided by participants in this study. While pain management was not brought up as an issue, some participants reported such issues as noise in the hallways, nursing activities that interfered with sleep and having to wait an inordinate amount of time for assistance with nausea. The collective tone of the narratives was that nurses were very busy, not that there was a discrepancy in the perception of needs. If care was not perceived, participants were quick to defend the nurse by acknowledging the nurses were too busy. In addition, participants felt the need to be protective of nurses' time, almost a reverse-caregiver role. Patients were aware of problems that impacted quality of life while in the hospital such as waiting for a nurse to respond to a call light, or perceptions of noise in the hallway that interfere with rest. Patients were also protective of nurses' time, and quick to offer excuses (lack of time) for issues that affected the patients' quality of life while in the hospital, such as inordinate noise and not responding in a timely manner.

The phenomenological study by Kralik et al (1997) considered what patients perceived as important about nursing care, and identified two major themes: engagement and detachment. Engagement was supported by the minor themes of nurses approaching the patient in such a manner that conveyed that nothing was too much trouble in their care, consulting with the patient, smiling and using humor, having the qualities of being kind and compassionate, knowing what was needed without having to be asked, being available, friendly, warm, and using a gentle touch. The theme of detachment was supported by such perceived behaviors as "treating the patient as a number" (depersonalization), being too efficient or busy, conveying that the patient should "try harder" or encouraging to the extreme, not sharing information with the patient, even when asked, having "rough hands", and approaching the job of nursing as "just a job" or "just doing what they are told". Similarly, Tumblin and Simkin (2001), Larrabee and Bolden (2001) and Radwin (2000) identified physical comfort, emotional support, providing instruction and information, attentiveness, coordination of activities, individualization and technical skills as expectations of the nurses' role by patients. Most of the behaviors identified by Kralik et al, Tumblin and Simkin, Larrabee and Bolden, and Radwin were also identified by the various participants in this study as elements of good nursing care. Individualization and "treating me as a human being", being seen as a unique individual, but also the commonality of being human, was repeatedly mentioned as exemplary of good nursing by participants in this study. However, participants did not identify all behaviors as having been exhibited by their nurses. Specifically, the concept that the nurse should convey that nothing is too much trouble in their care was not generally perceived. In fact, body language and demeanor of nurses toward the participants indicated that the nurses did not have time to be fully present. Participants believed they should be protective of the nurses' time because they did not want to trouble the nurses. Hewison (1995) described nurse/patient interaction as being superficial and routine, and suggested nurses had a 'power over' relationship with patients in their care. This superficiality is not conducive to communication or relationship building, and could explain in part the tendency of patients in the current study to believe they were infringing on nurses' time if they requested anything perceived to be outside the routine.

2. Are the Actions of Nurses to Address Spiritual Health Perceived by Patients as Fulfilling their Expectations?

Although not couched in the same terminology, participants in this study perceived actions that address spiritual health and described these actions in their descriptions of good nursing care. Conversely, actions that did not offer caring presence were often defining characteristics of bad nursing care. In their own experience of spiritual nursing care, participants generally believed that spiritual nursing care involved attending to religious aspects of spirituality. Although actions to address caring presence, 'being with', were certainly appreciated, they were not an expectation. In addition, actions to address any religious aspects of spiritual care on the part of the nurse, were not only not expected, they were often unwelcome, as indicated by Mary, who, as a devout Christian, did not want to be prayed for because "they might be praying for the wrong thing".

Spiritual care begins with presence (Burkhardt and Nagai-Jacobson, 2002) and is the basic way that spirituality is integrated into nursing care (Davidhizar et al., 2000). In addition, the spiritual component of presence has two distinct aspects, the existential qualities and actions such as kindness, touch empathy, and connectedness, and spirituality as expressed by religiosity to include religious rituals and prayer. The North American Nursing Diagnosis Association (NANDA) now recognizes the distinction between existential spirituality and religious spirituality, and has revised nursing diagnoses to reflect spirituality and religiosity separately (Burkhart, 2001).

Of note, although elements of both 'being there' and 'being with' were described as good nursing care by the study participants, and were certainly perceived by the participants, only physical presence, 'being there' was expected. Participants described the expectation of competence and watchfulness over physical needs as being important and a characteristic of good nursing. However, spiritual and psychological care, described in the 'being with' aspects of presence, was not an expectation. Participants described aspects of existential spiritual care, 'being with', such as touch, empathy, relatedness, eye contact, and kindness, as welcome and helpful, but not expected from the nurse. The aspects of 'being with' associated with religiosity, such as prayer, were expressly not expected, and in some cases, potentially detrimental, according to study participants.

Expectations are commonly based on experience. Participants expressed that the nurses were too busy or did not have time to do more than attend to physical needs. Hewison (1995) observed that most nurse/patient interaction was superficial, routine and talk-oriented and suggested that nurses had a 'power over' relationship with patients, which was a barrier to any meaningful communication between nurse and patient. Data generated by Hewison's study reflected that 'power over' and being treated in a routine manner as opposed to as an individual was indicative of bad nursing care. Indeed, some participants identified such behavior as indicative of bad nursing care. Perhaps this could be an explanation for participants in this study having no expectation of existential spiritual care, and emphatically not being desirous of any religious aspects of spiritual care. Because patients in the hospital have a sense of vulnerability, it would neither be expected nor wanted for anyone seen as having 'power over' to delve into anything that in essence defines them as a human being.

3. What Actions by Nurses are Perceived as Spiritual Interventions by Patients?

Spiritual interventions perceived by participants in this study were centered around the religious patterns of spirituality such as prayer or referral to clergy, and knowing when to make such referral. Activities of presence such as touching, exhibiting care and concern, communicating to include listening and explaining medical care, making the participant feel less vulnerable, and sharing of self were also perceived, but not necessarily labeled or recognized as being spiritual by participants. However, such activities were recognized as elements of "good" nursing care. One participant identified the act of caring to be spiritual and described such attributes as coaching and exhibiting humor as evidence of spiritual care from his nurse. This was consistent with the humanistic framework. The existential nature of care includes an element of reciprocity, meaning that what is conveyed should be perceived as being conveyed (Appleton, 1993; Burkhardt and Nagai-Jacobson, 2000; Patterson and Zderad, 1988; Taylor, 2002).

Touch was identified as conveying caring, connectedness and a sense of 'being with' by two participants. Results of the study conducted by Mulaik et al (1991) also indicated that patients viewed touch as indicative of caring and that touch by the nurses was important in care. The study by Mulaik et al also indicated that 59% of respondents also reported that touch indicated control on the part of the nurse and should not be used often. Although, specific questions about touch were not included in the current study, participants did not mention perceiving touch as a means of control.

Two qualitative studies (Concho, 1995 and Sellers, 2001) that addressed patient's perceptions of spiritual care described spiritual interventions consistent with those described in this study. Participants in both Sellers' and Conco's studies were self-identified as being Christian, and described establishing a caring relationship, presence, listening and giving of self (sharing) as included in effective nursing care. In addition, they reported that people feel connected to others who share the same spiritual beliefs and examining meaning or purpose in life was described as spiritual caregiving by participants. This finding was not borne out in the current study, which, via sampling for maximum variation, recruited both religious and nonreligious participants. While one participant in the current study reported finding comfort if she and the nurse had common religious beliefs, other participants reported not having any expectation of spiritual care, other than to be referred to clergy. In addition, one participant in the current study, an atheist, expressly did not want the religious aspects of spiritual care and objected to the word "spiritual". Of note, another participant, self-identified as Episcopalian, reported being leery of nurses who offer to pray for her because they may not share her specific religious beliefs and may pray for the wrong thing, even if they are Christians.

4. How do Individuals Define Spiritual Care?

Spiritual care was defined by participants in this study mainly in terms of religiosity – religious beliefs, prayer, needs provided by a minister, and connection to a higher power. Three individuals defined spiritual care as caring and went on to describe behaviors associated with nursing presence such as empathy, sympathy and "being there for you". Two participants specifically differentiated between religion and spirituality, identifying religion in terms of a belief pattern and spirituality in terms of nursing presence. These same concepts were identified by participants in the Sellers (2001) study, in which spiritual care was characterized as nurses understanding the unique human experience by establishing a caring relationship to include being present, listening, respecting and giving of self.

Conco (1995) reported that spiritual care was given when caregivers shared their own beliefs in a supreme being with the patients. This idea of sharing of beliefs was identified by two participants in this study, who went on to indicate that spiritual care as described by Conco would have been welcomed. As was also found in the current study, both Conco and Sellers reported spiritual care as having strong religious connotations. I found that spiritual care was defined by patients mainly in terms of religiosity, and is neither expected, nor desired, from nurses in the hospital. To a lesser extent, spiritual care was described by behaviors consistent with nursing presence as described in the literature.

Religious aspects of spirituality are addressed in the literature by studies using various Likert type questionnaires to describe or measure components of spirituality such as purpose in life, life salience, ego strength, self image, perceived well-being, religious orientation, and existential wellbeing (Ellison, 1983; McCutcheon, 1998; O'Neill and Kenny, 1998; Shek, 1991). Religious aspects of spirituality dominate the content of these questionnaires. In defining spirituality, participants in the current study also discussed some of the same concepts measured in the various questionnaires including belief systems, religious orientation and practices such as prayer, and meaning or purpose in life. However, the majority of participants defined spirituality in terms of religious affiliation, belief in a higher being, and religious practices such as prayer. They acknowledged that that which gave meaning or purpose to life could be important, but primarily, spirituality was synonymous with religiosity. Of note, those participants who self-identified as agnostic and atheistic identified spirituality in terms of religion as strongly, or more strongly than participants who self-identified as Christian. Other consistent themes included in definitions of spirituality were appreciating nature, music, taking time to determine what is meaningful to the patient, active listening, being with, sharing self, demonstrating that the patient was valued and seen as a human being, and connection to others and to a higher power.

Reker, Peacock and Wong (1981) and Drolet (1990) utilized questionnaires designed to explore concepts associated with spiritual beliefs such as life purpose, death acceptance and symbolic immortality. Interestingly, these concepts were not mentioned as elements of spirituality by participants in this study. On the other hand, no participant specifically excluded these concepts from spiritual beliefs either.

The defining characteristics of spiritual care are also consistent with definitions of spiritual care in the theoretical literature. Quantitative studies of spirituality have been conducted largely with regard to religiosity (Giblin,

1997; Reed, 1987; Richards, 1991). Spiritual care is often confused with, or used interchangeably with religiosity. Given that, spiritual needs are often referred to a chaplain or minister. Burkhart (2001), in her report for the Spirituality and Religiousness Diagnosis Working Group, North American Nursing Diagnosis Association (NANDA) acknowledged that, in clinical nursing, spiritual nursing care has historically been defined in terms of religious preference or practice. Recognizing that this conceptualization does not address patients who do not have religious affiliations, this working group developed separate definitions for spirituality and religiosity. The new definition of spirituality encompasses the concepts of purpose in life, connection to self, others and a higher being, art, music, literature and nature.

In summary, consistent with the literature, participants in this study defined spirituality primarily in terms of religiosity or religious practices such as prayer. Other experiences used to define spirituality included appreciating nature, music, taking time to determine what is meaningful to the patient, active listening, being with, sharing self, demonstrating that the patient was valued and seen as a human being, and connection to others and to a higher power.

Although the data generating strategy for this study was to achieve maximum variation in respondents, the majority of the respondents self-identified as Christian, limiting responses, particularly in defining spirituality, to those reflecting Christian belief systems. Even those participants self-identified as agnostic or atheistic responded based on their own knowledge base or background, which was in all cases, Christian. The resulting data was rich, but the particular perspectives of Islam, Judaism and Eastern teachings and beliefs were not represented and could further enrich the understanding of spirituality and spiritual care.

In addition, all the respondents were Caucasian. Even within the same religious belief system, here Christianity, there are a wide variety of interpretations and practices among different ethnic and cultural groups. That variability was not reflected in this participant group. Because both religious and spiritual practices are largely influenced by cultural and ethnic traditions, the lack of variability related to culture and ethnicity is a limitation of the current study, particularly in understanding the phenomena of spirituality and spiritual care.

Questions in this study related specifically to caring practices of nurses in a hospital setting. One of my assumptions was that the participants would respond truthfully. I have no reason to believe that participants did not respond truthfully during their interviews. However, because I was known to the participants to be a nurse, it is possible that the participants told me what they thought I wanted to hear.

Many hospitals in the United States have religious sponsorship or affiliations while others are secular for profit and not for profit institutions. I did not ask, nor was it apparent in the collection of data for this study if participants were hospitalized in religious or non-religious affiliated hospitals. Examining responses to the study questions and narrative stories in light of whether or not participants were hospitalized in a religious-based institution could have added to a deeper understanding of the phenomenon of patient expectations of spiritual care by their nurses.

RECOMMENDATIONS FOR FUTURE STUDIES

Further research is warranted to explore the concept of spiritual care as part of holistic nursing practice. Participants in this study were able to describe good and bad nursing care. Based on the responses of participants in this study, one of the most compelling conclusions I have reached with regard to spiritual care is that existential spiritual care is the hallmark of good nursing care. Conversely, lack of existential spiritual care was a definitive characteristic of bad nursing care. Clarifying and exploring the meaning of spiritual nursing care is therefore imperative in investigating quality nursing care practices and nursing education.

One of the potential limitations of this study, was that a nurse conducted the interviews, and participants responses were influenced by that fact. It is equally possible that participants were more considered in their responses because a nurse cared enough to ask questions about their hospitalizations. To address the potential for biased responses, either positive or negative, during the course of the interview, a non-nurse researcher could ask the interview questions. Comparisons could be drawn between responses elicited by a nurse, as in this study, and those elicited in a future study by a non-nurse. Hypothetically, responses elicited by the non-nurse researcher should be comparable to those elicited by the nurse researcher.

The lack of variability related to cultural and ethnic traditions is a possible limitation of the current study. Both religious and spiritual practices are largely influenced by cultural and ethnic traditions. Although one participant was atheistic and two were agnostic, the religious and cultural traditions of all participants in this study were Christian-based. It would be appropriate to address spiritual care perceptions through the lens of cultural and ethnic traditions. It would also be interesting to solicit respondents with more diverse religious backgrounds. It would also be exciting to explore perceptions of spiritual care among children of various developmental levels.

Spiritual care perceptions in this study were investigated from the perspective of the patient. Having a better understanding of the expectations regarding care in general and spiritual care specifically from the perspective of the patient, it seems logical to interview nurses regarding their perceptions of the care they provide, to include spiritual aspects of care. It would be interesting to present the findings of this study to a focus group of practicing nurses and discuss practice implications. Within the framework of humanistic nursing, there should be no difference in the perceptions of spiritual care between nurse respondents and patient respondents. In addition, nurses descriptions of exemplary nursing characteristics should parallel the characteristics of good nurses as described by the participants in the current study

Many scientific studies have been conducted that indicate there is a relationship between stress and the immune system. Does spiritual caregiving have a measurable effect on stress? Do religious beliefs or lack of a belief system have an effect on stress or perception of stress? Given that there is a measureable effect of stress on the immune system, if stress is ameliorated by spiritual care, the immune system would be enhanced. On the other hand, if stress is exacerbated by a lack of or inappropriate spiritual care, the immune system would be weakened. Religiosity of the patient may have a similar effect on stress perception and therefore the immune system. A future study could be conducted exploring the relationship between spirituality and religiosity, stress, and the immune system.

CONCLUSION

This study resulted in several interesting findings. First, nursing presence was seen by patients as important and elements of nursing presence were used to describe good nursing care. 'Being there', with elements of nursing competence (knowing what is going on and technical proficiency), as well as nursing surveillance (keeping track, notifying physicians as warranted, watching carefully), was a universal expectation of nurses. 'Being with', the existential spiritual element of presence (kindness, gentleness, caring touch) was the most defining characteristic of good nursing care as described by participants, but was not expected. Sharing of self, and element of existential spiritual care is generally discouraged in my experience as a nurse, both in nursing schools and in hospital settings, but was clearly appreciated from the patients' perspective. All participants were able to define spirituality, most frequently in terms of religiosity and religious practices such as prayer. Spiritual nursing care was most frequently described as recognizing the need to refer the patient to a minister. The religious element of spirituality was not expected or wanted, by some, adamantly.

Time was a strong recurrent theme. Perceptions of nursing not having time (scurrying in the hallways, not talking to the patient when in the room, not making eye contact) were mentioned by 9 of the 11 participants. Perceiving the nurses as too busy led to patients not requesting care. This perceived lack of time was then offered as a reason for not expecting existential spiritual care. Sourial (1997) concluded that nurses viewed physical care was an imperative, whereas psychosocial or existential care was only provided if there was time. This is consistent with study participant's perceptions.

The framework for investigating the concept of time with relation to patient care is provided in the theory of humanistic nursing (Pattrson and Zderad, 1988). Humanistic nursing recognizes that, in the transactional nature of nursing, there is an intersubjectivity between nurse and patient that results in a timing of behaviors aimed at developing the patient's human potential. In general, the findings of this study were congruent with the literature with the exception of patient expectations of spiritual interventions by their nurse. In addition, the theoretical framework of humanistic nursing was appropriate to describe the phenomenon of spiritual care and supports continued analysis and implementation of spiritual care.

The research questions of this study were addressed in the narratives of the participants. Findings of this study contribute to the understanding of the role of the nurse in providing spiritual care within a holistic nursing care framework. The opportunity to continue to research spiritual care, to include clarifying and reinforcing spiritual dimensions of care as it relates to individuals and to populations is illuminated.

REFERENCES

Adamsen, L. and Tewes, M. (2000). Discrepancy between patients' perspectives, staff's documentation and reflections on basic nursing care. *Scandinavian Journal of Caring Science,* 14, 120-129.

Appleton, C. (1993). The art of nursing: The experience of patients and nurses. *Journal of Advanced Nursing, 18,* 892-899.

Benner, P. (1985). Quality of life: A phenomenological perspective on explanation, prediction, and understanding in nursing science. *Advances in Nursing Science, 8(1),* 1-14.

Bensley, R. (1991). Defining spiritual health: A review of the literature. *Journal of Health Education,* 22(5), 287-290.

Bohm, D. (Ed. Nichol, L.) (1996). *On dialogue.* New York: Routledge, Taylor and Francis Group.

Brush, B. and Daly, P. (2000). Assessing spirituality in primary care practice: Is there time? *Clinical Excellence for Nurse Practitioners,* 4(2), 67-71.

Burkhardt, M. (1989). Spirituality: An analysis of the concept. *Holistic Nursing Practice,* 3(3), 69-77.

Burkhardt, M. and Nagai-Jacobson, M. (2002). *Spirituality: Living our connectedness.* Albany, NY: Delmar.

Burkhart, L. (2001). Notes on NDEC: Report from the spirituality and religiousness diagnosis working group. *Nursing Diagnosis,* 12(2), 61062.

Carroll, B. (2001). A phenomenological exploration of the nature of spirituality and spiritual care. *Mortality,* 6(1), 81-99.

Carson, V. (1989). *Spiritual dimensions of nursing practice.* Philadelphia: W.B. Saunders Co.

Chase-Ziolck, M. and Gruca, J. (2000). Clients' perceptions of distinctive aspects in nursing care received within a congregational setting. *Journal of Community Health Nursing,* 17(3), 171-183.

Clarke, J. and Wheeler, S. (1992). A view of the phenomenon of caring in nursing practice. *Journal of Advanced Nursing, 17,* 1283-1290.

Concho, D. (1995). Christian patients' view of spiritual care. *Western Journal of Nursing Research, 17(3),*266-277.

Cortis, J. (2000). Caring as experienced by minority ethnic patients. *International Nursing Review,* 47(1), 53-63.

Cumbie, S. (2001). The integration of mind-body-soul and the practice of humanistic nursing. *Holistic Nursing Practice,* 15(3), 56-62.

Davidhizar, R, Bechtel, G, and Cosey, E. (2000). The spiritual needs of hospitalized patients. *American Journal of Nursing,* 100(7), 24C-24D.

Davis, L. (2005). A phenomenological study of patient expectations concerning nursing care. *Holistic Nursing Practice, 19(3),* 126-133.

Dossey, B. (1998). Holistic modalities and healing moments. *American Journal of Nursing,* 98(6), 44-47.

Dossey, B. and Dossey, L. (1998). Body-mind-spirit: Attending to holistic care. *American Journal of Nursing*, 98(8), 35-38.

Drain, M. (2001). Quality improvement in primary care and the importance of patient perceptions. *Journal of Ambulatory Care Management,* 24(2), 30-46.

Drolet, J. (1990). Transcending death during early adulthood: Symbolic immortality, death anxiety, and purpose in life. *Journal of Clinical Psychology,* 46(2), 148-160.

Dyson, J., Cobb, M., and Forman, D. (1997). The meaning of spirituality: A literature review. *Journal of Advanced Nursing*, 26, 1183-1188.

Ellison, C. (1983). Spiritual well-being: Conceptualization and measurement. *Journal of Psychology and Theology,* 11(4), 330-340.

Eriksson, E. (2001). Caring for cancer patients: Relatives' assessments of received care. *European Journal of Cancer Care,* 10(1), 48-56.

Erlandson, D., Harris, E., Skipper, B., and Allen, S. (1993). *Doing naturalistic inquiry: A guide to methods.* Newbury Park: SAGE Publications.

Espland, K. (1999). Achieving spiritual wellness: Using reflective questions. *Journal of Psychosocial Nursing*, 37(7), 36-40.

Fagerstrom, L., Eriksson, K., and Engberg, I. (1999). The patient's perceived caring needs: Measuring the unmeasurable. *International Journal of Nursing Practice,* 5, 199-208.

Fontaine, K. (2000). *Healing practices: Alternative therapies for nursing.* Upper saddle River, NJ: Prentice Hall.

Frank, A. (1991). *At the will of the body: Reflections on illness.* Boston: Houghton Mifflin Company.

Frankl, V. (1984). *Man's search for meaning: An introduction to logotherapy.* New York: Simon and Schuster.

Fredriksson, L. (1999). Modes of relating in a caring conversation: A research synthesis on presence, touch and listening. *Journal of Advanced Nursing*, 30(5), 1167-1176.

Gilbin, P. (1997). Marital spirituality: A quantitative study. *Journal of Religion and Health*, 36(4), 321-332.

Giorgi, A. (1970). *Psychology as a human science: A phenomenologically based approach.* New York: Harper and Row.

Godkin, J. (2001). Healing presence. *Journal of Holistic Nursing.* 19(1), 5-21.

Halldorsdottir, S. and Hamrin, E. (1997). Caring and uncaring encounters within nursing and health care from the cancer patient's perspective. *Cancer Nursing, 20(2),* 120-128.

Hewison, A. (1995). Nurses' power in interactions with patients. *Journal of Advanced Nursing, 21*, 75-82.

Howard, B. and Howard, J. (1997). Occupation as spiritual activity. *The American Journal of Occupational Therapy*, 51(3), 181-185.

Kralik, D., Koch, T., and Wotton, K. (1997). Engagement and detachment: Understanding patients' experiences with nursing. *Journal of Advanced Nursing*, 26, 399-407.

Larrabee, J. and Bolden, L. (2001). Defining patient-perceived quality of nursing care. *Journal of Nursing Care Quality,* 16(1), 34-57.

Latham, C. (2001). Predictors of patient outcomes following interactions with nurses. *Western Journal of Nursing Research,* 18(5), 548-564.

McCutcheon, L. (1998). Life role salience scales: Additional evidence for construct validation. *Psychological Reports*, 83, 1307-1314.

McKinnon, N. (1991). Humanistic nursing: It can't stand up to scrutiny. *Nursing and Health Care*, 12(8), 414-416.

McSherry, W, and Draper, P. (1998). The debates emerging from the literature surrounding the concept of spirituality as applied to nursing. *Journal of Advanced Nursing*, 27(4), 683-691.

Meraviglia, M. (1999). Critical analysis of spirituality and its empirical indicators. *Journal of Holistic Nursing,* 17(1), 18-33.

Miles, M. and Huberman, A. (1994). *An expanded sourcebook: Qualitative data analysis.* Thousand Oaks, CA: SAGE Publications.

Mulaik, J., Megenity, J., Cannon, R., Chance, K., Cannella, K., Garland, L, and Gilead, M. (1991). Patients' perceptions of nurses' use of touch. *Western Journal of Nursing Research,* 13(3), 306-323.

Mulholland, J. (1995). Nursing, humanism and transcultural theory: The 'bracketing out' of reality. *Journal of Advanced Nursing,* 22(3), 442-449.

Nelms, T. (1996). Living a caring presence in nursing: A Heideggerian analysis. *Journal of Advanced Nursing,* 24(2), 368-374.

Newman, M. (1989). The spirit of nursing. *Holistic Nursing Practice*, 3(3), 1-6.

O'Neill, D, and Kenny, E. (1998). Spirituality and chronic illness. *Image: Journal of Nursing Scholarship*, 30(3), 275-280.

Patterson, E. (1998). The philosophy and physics of holistic health care: spiritual healing as a workable interpretation. *Journal of Advanced Nursing,* 27(2), 287-293.

Patterson, J. and Zderad, L. (1988). *Humanistic nursing.* New York: National League for Nursing.

Polkinghorne, D. (1988). *Narrative knowing and the human sciences.* Albany: State University of New York Press.

Quinn, J. (2000). The self as healer: Reflections from a nurse's journey. *AACN Clinical Issues: Advanced Practice in Acute Critical Care, 11(1),* 17-26.

Radwin, L. (2000). Oncology patients' perceptions of quality nursing care, *Research in Nursing Health,* 23, 179-190.

Reed, P. (1987). Spirituality and well-being in terminally ill hospitalized adults. *Research in Nursing and Health*, 10, 335-344.

Reed, P. (1992). An emerging paradigm for the investigation of spirituality in nursing. *Research in Nursing and Health*, 15, 349-357.

Reker, G., Peacock, E., and Wong, P. (1987). Meaning and purpose in life and well-being: A life-span perspective. *Journal of Gerontology*, 42(1), 44-49.

Richards, P. (1991). Religious devoutness in college students: Relations with emotional adjustment and psychological separation from parents. *Journal of Counseling Psychology*, 38(2), 189-196.

Ross, L. (1994). Spiritual aspects of nursing. *Journal of Advanced Nursing*, 19, 439-447.

Rogers, M. (1972). Nursing: To be or not to be? *Nursing Outlook*, 20(1), 42-46.

Sellers, S. (2001). The spiritual care meanings of adults residing in the Midwest. *Nursing Science Quarterly,* 14(3), 239-248.

Shek, D. (1991). Meaning in life and psychological well-being: An empirical study using the Chinese version of the Purpose in Life Questionnaire. *The Journal of Genetic Psychology*, 153(2), 185-200.

Sheldon, J. (2000). Spirituality as a part of nursing. *Journal of Hospice and Palliative Nursing,* 2(3), 101-108.

Sourial, S. (1997). An analysis of caring. *Journal of Advanced Nursing,* 26, 1189-1192.

Stranahan, S. (2001). Spiritual perception, attitudes about spiritual care, and spiritual care practice among nurse practitioners. *Western Journal of Nursing Research,* 23(1), 90-105.

Streubert, H. and Carpenter, D. (1999). *Qualitative research in nursing: Advancing the humanistic imperative.* Philadelphia: Lippincott.

Stuart, E., Deckro, J., and Mandle, C. (1989). Spirituality in health and healing: A clinical program. *Holistic Nursing Practice,* 3(3), 35-46.

Swanson, K. (1999). What is known about caring in nursing science: A literary meta-analysis. In A.S. Hinshaw, S. Feetham, and J. Shaver (Eds.), *Handbook of clinical nursing research* (pp. 31- 60). Thousand Oaks, CA: SAGE Publications.

Tanyi, R. (2002). Towards clarification of the meaning of spirituality. *Journal of Advanced Nursing, 39(5),* 500-509.

Taylor, E. (2002). *Spiritual care: Nursing theory, research, and practice.* Upper Saddle river, NJ: Prentice Hall.

Thomas, S. and Pollio, H. (2002). *Listening to patients: A phenomenological approach to nursing research and practice.* New York: Springer Publishing Company.

Travelbee, J. (1969). *Intervention in psychiatric nursing: Process in the one-to-one relationship.* Philadelphia: FA Davis.

Tumblin, A. and Simkin, P. (2001). Pregnant women's perceptions of their nurse's role during labor and delivery. *Perinatal Care,* 28(1), 52-56.

Van der Zalm, J. and Bergum, V. (2000). Hermeneutic-phenomenology: providing living knowledge for nursing practice. *Journal of Advanced Nursing,* 31(1), 211-218.

Van Manen, M. (1990). *Researching lived experiences.* London, Ontario: State University of New York Press.

Watson, J. (1985). *Nursing: The philosophy and science of caring.* Niwot, CO: The University Press of Colorado.

Watson, J. (1999). Postmodern nursing and beyond. New York: Churchill Livingstone.

Watson, J. and Smith, M (2002). Caring science and the science of unitary human beings: A trans-theoretical discourse for nursing knowledge development. *Journal of Advanced Nursing, 37(5),* 452-461.

Woolf, H (Ed.). (1975). *Webster's new collegiate dictionary* (6th ed.). Springfield MA: GandC Merriam Co.

Wright, K. (1998). Professional, ethical and legal implications for spiritual care in nursing. *Image: Journal of Nursing Scholarship*, 30, 1, 82-83.

In: Religion and Healthcare   ISBN 978-1-61324-256-8
Editors: A.M. Curtis and D.P. Werthel   © 2012 Nova Science Publishers, Inc.

Chapter 3

FAITH-BASED SUBSTANCE ABUSE TREATMENT PROGRAMS

Amy W. Dominguez, Chin-Chin Ip, David Hoover,
Ariel Oleari, Mark R. McMinn, Tracy W. Lee,
Nicole L. Steiner-Pappalardo and Miral Luka
Wheaton College IL, U.S.A.

As spirituality and religiousness are gaining attention as important
variables in health care and psychological well being, it is timely to consider
the religious and spiritual aspects of treatment for substance abuse as well.
Faith-based substance-abuse treatment programs are explored through both
quantitative and qualitative measures in efforts to understand the specific
ways these programs incorporate components of client's faith with sound
mental health treatment, hoping to learn about specific models of faith-based
substance abuse treatment.

One of the most troubling and persistent challenges in the field of psychology is the gulf between research and practice. Greenberg (1994) laments, "the two groups are separated virtually from professional birth" (p. 1). This estrangement has various consequences, ranging from a major split within the American Psychological Association (APA)—resulting in the formation of the American Psychological Society (APS)—to disputes about the practical relevance of empirically validated treatment procedures (Crits-Christoph, Chambless, Frank, Brody, and Karp, 1995; Garfield, 1996; Havik and VandenBos, 1996; Silverman, 1996).

Perhaps paradoxically, acknowledging a gap between science and practice demonstrates a desire to keep them together. Indeed, most clinical psychologists identify themselves as both scientists and practitioners, and a number of researchers and clinicians are investing significant effort in bridging the gap between research and practice (e.g., Norcross, 2002; Talley, Strupp, and Butler, 1994).

As spirituality and religion are gaining attention as important variables for psychological inquiry and health promotion—evidenced by a growing number of journal articles and books published by the APA (Hill and Pargament, 2003; Miller, 1999; Miller and Thoresen, 2003; Powell, Shahabi, and Thoresen, 2003; Richards and Bergin, 1997, 2000, 2004; Seeman, Dubin, and Seeman, 2003; Shafranske, 1996)—it is important to consider the integration of science and practice in relation to spiritual interventions. This need is highlighted by a recent review of the substance abuse outcome literature.

Lee, Luka, McMinn, Dominguez, and Steiner-Pappalardo (2004) conducted an evaluation of the 12-step recovery literature in which they located 104 published and unpublished outcome studies. They found only a minority of outcome studies assessed clients' religious beliefs or behaviors. Even those few studies that make some effort at religious or spiritual assessment are likely to do so by asking one particular question (e.g., denominational affiliation) and then often fail to include the religious variable when reporting results. This is particularly surprising when considering the central role of spirituality in 12-step recovery programs. Lee et al. (2004) conclude that there is something like a science/practice split when it comes to spirituality and 12-step programs.

The split may go even deeper than science and practice, revealing a gulf between prevailing standards of care in mental health professions and the ministry concerns of spiritual practitioners. When recovery programs emerged in the 1930s, they began with an intentional spiritual emphasis. Decades later, much of this emphasis on spirituality has dissipated, at least among the programs rooted in psychological science. This leaves a bifurcated state of affairs: on the one hand, mental health practitioners have few, if any, explicitly religious or spiritual programs that focus on treating substance abuse; on the other hand, religious communities and individuals have substance abuse treatment programs that may have little footing in the standards of empirically-based mental health care. Thus, the two studies reported here represent a beginning effort to assess the apparent gulf between substance abuse treatment programs rooted in psychological science and recovery programs within religious communities. The first study explored clergy attitudes and experiences with substance abuse problems in their parishes, using a general survey methodology. We also assessed what resources clergy rely upon with parishioners who wrestle with substance abuse. The second study involved telephone interviews designed to better understand the spiritual and psychological methods and practices of faith-based substance abuse programs.

STUDY 1

Method

A sample of 376 clergy in Illinois was randomly identified from church listings at gtesuperpages.com to receive a questionnaire. To ensure a representative sample of denominations, clergy were selected from 69 categories (e.g., Anglican, Baptist, Catholic, Eastern Orthodox, Korean). Contact information was gathered from the web site. Churches were phoned to obtain as many pastors' names as possible, in order to personalize the mailing. Questionnaires were mailed to 376 clergy along with a $2 incentive in appreciation for their participation. One hundred forty-one (141) clergy responded with completed questionnaires and 26 were not deliverable, resulting in an overall response rate of 40%. Of the 141 who responded, 85% were male and 15% were female. Most respondents (83%) were European American, 11% were African American, 4% were Asian or Asian American, and 2% did not indicate their ethnicity. Clergy respondents, on the average, were 49 years old (ranging from 27 to 93), had been in church service for 21 years (ranging from 1 to 55 years), had been at their present church for 10 years (ranging from 1 to 52 years), and reported 318 as the average attendance at weekly worship services (ranging from 11 to 3000). Most of the completed questionnaires were filled out by the senior pastor (85%), 7% by an associate pastor, 4% by a church leader, 1% by a church secretary, and 3% did not indicate the position of the respondent in the church.

We constructed the questionnaire to gather information regarding how churches are encountering and addressing those struggling with substance abuse. Additionally, we wanted to gain an understanding about what is being done in various churches and what support may be needed to strengthen Christian communities. The questionnaire consisted of three sections: 1) About you and your ministry; 2) Making decisions about substance abuse problems; and 3) Responding to substance abuse problems. The first section included demographic information, frequency of encounters with those seeking help for substance abuse problems, and general opinions of the respondents regarding the etiology of substance abuse. The second section addressed the response of the church and staff to those with substance abuse problems as well as available resources. The third section queried about the recovery approach of the church and the degree of satisfaction with the outcomes resulting from these approaches. We then asked open-ended questions regarding sources of assistance in a crisis situation and specifically Christian resources that may be available in the immediate community of the respondents. Additional comments were invited as well.

Results and Discussion

We asked respondents a series of questions regarding how they make decisions when confronting substance abuse problems in their congregations. They rated each of the items on a Likert scale ranging from 1 (strongly disagree) to 5 (strongly agree). Results are summarized in Table 1.

It was clear from the findings that pastors would like to have resources within the church to handle substance abuse problems internally (i.e., they do not want to rely exclusively on referring people outside the church), but most do not perceive that they have ample resources within their congregation to address substance abuse problems when they occur. Most churches make case-by-case decisions rather than having specific policies or treatment models in place to handle substance abuse problems, and most do not have a specific person designated to handle substance abuse problems when they arise.

We tested for group differences, using a liberal .05 alpha level because of the exploratory nature of this research. Males were more likely than females to say that substance abuse problems should be handled outside the church, F (1, 123) = 4.5, $p < .05$. Ethnicity differences were also observed on the degree to which respondents were aware of treatment resources available in the community, F (3, 125) = 2.7, $p < .05$. Post-hoc contrasts using Least Squared Differences tests revealed that European Americans reported greater awareness of resources than African American, $p < .05$, or Asian American respondents, $p < .05$. Correlational analyses revealed that the age of pastors is positively related to the extent they report that substance abuse should be handled outside the church, $r = .27, p < .01$. Also, the length of time a pastor has been at the church is positively related to the church having a specific plan for handling substance abuse cases, $r = .21, p < .05$. The size of the congregation is positively correlated with the likelihood of making case-by-case decisions, $r = .20, p < .05$ and having a specific policy, $r = .17, p < .05$.

Table 1. Decision-Making when Faced with Substance Abuse Problems

Item	N	Mean	S.D.	Group Differences
We choose not to respond, because helping with substance abuse is best handled outside the church.	140	1.6	0.8	Males endorsed more than females.
We discuss how to handle it among the leadership team.	136	3.1	1.2	
We designate one person to handle these matters.	138	2.3	1.3	
We make case-by-case decisions as the need arises.	137	4.1	1.1	
We have a specific policy for handling substance abuse problems.	139	2.3	1.2	
We are satisfied with how we are helping people with substance abuse problems.	136	2.8	1.1	
We are satisfied with the recovery resources available to us in the community.	138	2.9	1.1	
We have ample resources within our church to address substance abuse problems.	141	2.2	1.1	
We have a treatment model for addressing substance abuse problems in our church.	140	2.2	1.2	
We are aware of what resources are available in the community.	141	3.8	1.0	European Americans endorsed this item more than African Americans or Asian Americans.
Many people in the congregation are aware of resources available in the community.	140	3.1	1.0	

We also asked what sort of treatment approaches pastors recommend for those facing substance abuse problems. For each of the 7 options listed in Table 2 we asked what percentage of substance abuse cases they handled this way and then asked them to rate their satisfaction with this approach on a Likert scale ranging from 1 (not at all) to 5 (a great deal). Spiritual interventions are by far the most common, followed by pastoral counseling, peer accountability within the church, and referral to a counselor outside the church. Satisfaction ratings for each of these approaches are modest, hovering around the midpoint of the 5-point Likert scale. Because many respondents did not complete the items on this part of the questionnaire, thereby making some ethnic and gender groups too small for group comparisons, we were not able to test for group differences.

Table 2. Treatment Approaches

Item	Percentage of Cases Handled this Way			Satisfaction with the Outcome		
	N	Mean	S.D.	N	Mean	S.D.
Spiritual direction (e.g., prayer, scripture, guidance, fasting).	117	75.0	34.3	107	3.6	1.0
Recommend reading and audiovisual materials.	104	37.1	35.3	81	2.8	1.0
Peer accountability within the church.	110	47.2	37.2	90	3.4	1.1
Pastoral counseling within the church.	113	56.0	34.3	98	3.4	0.9
Support group within the church.	91	31.0	38.6	58	2.9	1.5
Referral to a counselor outside the church.	108	47.8	36.5	93	3.4	1.1
Referral to a support group outside the church.	100	41.3	37.1	87	3.2	1.2

Throughout the questionnaire we asked respondents to identify particular resources they have found useful when parishioners face substance abuse problems. A wide variety of agencies, professional counselors, support groups, and treatment centers were identified. Although 14 different church-based support groups were identified, Alcoholics Anonymous (AA) was the only such group mentioned by more than one respondent. Ten respondents mentioned AA groups in their churches. Similarly, 14 different support groups outside the church were useful to respondents, but Teen Challenge and AA were the only outside groups identified by more than one respondent. Four respondents mentioned Teen Challenge and 35 identified AA. When asked about Christian resources for substance abuse, many respondents identified particular therapists, books, or programs but Teen Challenge was the only one identified by more than a few respondents. Teen Challenge was mentioned by 7 of our clergy respondents.

Respondents' beliefs about the etiology of substance abuse were also assessed. These results are not relevant to this particular investigation, and are reported elsewhere (Dominguez, McMinn, Lee, Luka, and Steiner-Pappalardo, 2003).

STUDY 2

Methods

Early in 2004, 97 faith-based substance abuse treatment centers were contacted. Clergy (from Study 1) had referenced some of these programs while others were found through other sources, including the Internet. These potential information sources were each called at least once, some several times, to arrange for interviewing. Of these programs, 15 participated in a 20-minute recorded phone interview. Interviewers gathered information about the programs' organizational development, types and structure of service provision, clients served, funding, credentials, integrative approach, treatment model, effectiveness data, and aftercare. Interviews were coded and analyzed using N6, a qualitative software coding program.

We constructed the interview to better understand the particular ways that faith-based treatment programs are incorporating faith issues with mental health treatment. Additionally, we wanted to gain an understanding about what is being done in various programs to inform clinicians and those interested in future program development. The interview consisted of 32 questions (most were open-ended) divided among 7 sections: organizational issues, credentials, clients, fees, follow up, service provision, and integrative approach. These 7 sections can be clustered into three broader categories: organization, services, and treatment model.

Organization

We asked for information relevant to the development of the specific organization, inquiring into the presence of a known mission statement (and, if one is used, the particular ways in which the program is carrying out this mission), the goals of the agency (current and future), and organizational challenges. In addition, information was gathered regarding the credentials of the agency, such as licensing information, staff training, and professional endorsements received by the agency.

Services

We also inquire about the nature of the services provided (e.g., evaluation, general consultation, individual therapy, group therapy, referral, or continuing education), program structure (i.e., residential, outpatient, etc. and corresponding frequency, i.e. daily, weekly, etc.), as well as the population served, intake and referral information, methods of service marketing, client fees, funding, aftercare, perceived efficacy of the program, methods of assessing effectiveness, and longitudinal data.

Treatment Model

We were also interested in the integrative nature of the program and the degree of perceived efficacy with the outcomes resulting from these approaches. We asked about the agency's approach to care, the ways in which faith issues are explored, the specific models of faith-incorporation employed, how mental health treatment is provided, and the specific treatment models used.

Results and Discussion

During the interview process, it quickly became evident that there is great variety in what is referred to as faith-based treatment. Two main variables emerged, around which programs may be categorized based on program concentrations: Faith Emphasis and Mental Health Emphasis. A subcategory also emerged in both areas: Basic Needs Emphasis. While most programs fit neatly into either a Faith Emphasis or Mental Health Emphasis conceptualization, several programs presented their approach as a unique amalgamation of the two main emphases.

Basic Needs Emphasis

Some programs are intent on addressing basic needs, such as physical needs, housing, medical needs, legal assistance, vocational needs, educational needs, and operating at low cost (or no cost) to participants. This type of focus varied among the programs and across both the faith and mental health emphases.

Faith Emphasis

Three programs interviewed view supporting participants' faith through Biblical care as the primary emphasis, excluding all explicit mental health models and materials unless they are directly compatible with scripture. Developing a personal relationship with Christ is emphasized through the structure of the programs, such as providing Bible teaching in daily chapel services, incorporating prayer and devotional time into daily life, mandating Bible class participation, and providing individual Biblical counsel and prayer. Clients come largely from word-of-mouth referrals, or through churches or other ministry settings.

Funding seems to be a main challenge with these ministries (they are funded largely by donations), followed by providing encouragement to clients, and staffing needs. These ministries have staff that have participated in Christian-based recovery (most are graduates of the same program in which they work), they view character change through Christ as essential, and anything that does not lead to such, unnecessary. One cited as the guiding verse for that agency as, "What should profit a man if he gains everything and loses his soul?" These staff have received the very same type of assistance they offer, that which leads others to know Christ and to become new people in Him.

Highly structured, stringent, accountability-focused, and long-term in nature (1 year minimum), these programs boast great success rates for participants who are able to complete them, though much of this is based on anecdotal information. These programs maintain a deep care for basic needs and addressed such in their work, evidenced in offering educational assistance, job training, long term housing opportunities, training which stresses post-program transitional success, and low or no cost services to participants. Follow up is stressed, and efforts are made to keep in touch with graduates of these programs.

Mental Health Emphasis

These six programs have varied approaches to care, all of which use traditional AA models, along with approaches such as brief therapy, biogenetic approaches, medication, detoxification and stabilization, drug and alcohol education, and all levels of therapy. Settings include inpatient and partial hospital, private practice, and community agencies. They are funded through insurance or self-pay. These programs have trained staff (i.e., Certified Alcohol and Drug Counselors, Master's level therapists, psychiatrists, and psychologists) working for them. Referrals come from the telephone book, insurance companies, courts, or other clients. Challenges for this group were systemic, from frustrations related to insurance to "internal, bureaucratic havoc within DCFS."

While all identified their programs as addressing faith issues, they each did so one of two ways. Either they remained purposefully subtle, with interviewees professing a Christian faith but not talking about it unless a client asked, or they presented as quite vague, embracing all types of spirituality, while ignoring distinctly Christian concepts of God—for example, using classic AA, with the language of a "higher power," or being open to any or no religious practice whatsoever. One interviewee stated their program was faith-focused because the staff all meditate together every morning during their staff meeting. Recovery was not necessarily related to a client's faith, and they could recover from substance abuse without addressing faith issues at all if they so desire.

Several of these programs maintained a primary emphasis on basic care needs and individuation, structured to assist the recovering addict in "returning to a life of dignity and purpose so they can have goals for their life." One particular program offers participants "a safe environment for rest, study, prayer, and work that will bring spiritual and emotional healing." Some other ways basic care needs are emphasized include educational assistance, program-funding assistance, transitional living arrangements, life skills training, recovery literature, and parenting instruction.

Blending of Faith and Mental Health Emphases

Six programs maintained high attention to both faith and mental health issues in their participants' recovery, all the while focusing on supporting clients' basic needs as well. Each of these agencies blended aspects of Christian faith and mental health principles into their approaches to care, in different ways, but with several striking similarities that became apparent upon closer examination.

Each of these programs began in a similar way, by an individual responding to a personal burden or feeling led by God. Challenges faced by these programs are predominantly financial (none of these programs are government funded), affecting staff needs and space constraints. These are not typical mental health centers; rather, they are residential ministry centers (except for one which is not residential), so insurance does not cover treatment.

Of the six, 3 of these programs do not charge participants. One requests that only a client's medical fees, including medication costs, are paid ($40-

50/month), one charges approximately $375/month if a client has an income, and the last program can accept insurance for outpatient groups offered. Additional program funds come from individuals, churches, grants, fundraising, and a participant-run thrift store.

Staff range in training, including ministry-focused interns close to completion of an undergraduate degree, chaplains with master's degrees in counseling, certified and/or licensed drug and addictions counselors, and people who have been through the very recovery programs in which they work. One interviewee reported that 14 of their 18 staff were recovered graduates of that program, with little or no education beyond a high school diploma. He cited this as a weakness of their agency.

> We hope staff training in counseling skills will really increase success rates, as guys can really feel as though they not only developed a relationship with Christ but that they have dealt with the issues of their abuse. The fundamentalists would say you are compromising, and the learned world would say that you are some kind of fanatical Christian, but you gotta find that niche in between.

Other than these similar beginnings and funding needs, some commonalities evident among these programs can be categorized by the following: 1) they each maintained a high level of value for their participants' individual faith journeys, but without sacrificing their programs' explicitly Christian presentation, 2) each program upholds faith development as the ultimate goal, believing that the deeper level changes occur when relationship with God is addressed, 3) these programs incorporate principles from psychology and mental health research to support their work, and 4) these six maintain a focus on the participant in context, addressing both short- and longer-term needs.

Respecting others' faith while presenting Christianity. All of these programs are explicitly Christian. They do not present this in vague ambiguity nor do they await a client-led inquiry in order to discuss their faith. One interviewee explains,

> Before they come, they understand that we are a Christian-based drug and alcohol recovery program... we tell them that they are going to start each day with prayer and meditation and we read from the book of Proverbs for an hour each morning. We don't force Christ down their throat in the beginning because we want to get them used to the wisdom of God, introduce them

slowly. But they understand that that it is Christian based, so attendance to a church of their choice is mandatory.

Another program reports, "At assessment, we say we are a faith program explicit to God and Jesus Christ. They have to at least be open to that." In addition, all of these programs maintained a high respect for whatever faith a participant presents.

Encouragement of faith development as primary source for healing. Each of these particular faith-based substance abuse treatment programs also place primary emphasis upon an individual's faith development, specifically from a Christian perspective. One self-describes as, "explicitly Christian, we deal with issues spiritually, on the heart level, through building on a relationship with Christ, and if they don't have one we have them start there, checking their spiritual foundation" while another program provides a faith-based care on a "wide spectrum, from basic sharing of the gospel to intense discipleship, depending on the individual." One program provides uses this distinct strategy for faith- based treatment: "We have found the best approach is to present the Gospel, and to give the option of one other thing (chapel services, 12-step groups, other support groups, etc.). Most people end up going to the church." Another ministry describes guiding participants along gently and remembering the larger goal of their work. After receiving teaching on the 12-steps as they correspond to Scripture, they:

> assist people who are giving their life for the first time to Christ, we help them consider baptism... Although the walk on this world may not always be pretty, because we have the propensity to relapse, we offer them the chance for eternal life.

Drawing on aspects of psychological treatment. These programs, which blend faith and an understanding of mental health, use varied principles from the field of psychology, borrowing from such theories as cognitive, behavioral, client-centered, rational emotive therapy, rational recovery, and aspects of 12-step models. All of these who use 12-step models limit their use to certain concepts or components of a modified, explicitly Christian version of the steps. Each of these six programs also maintains openness to biological influences and corresponding treatment.

Several programs use cognitive and behavioral techniques in their treatment approach. One program's approach to care is summed up in their "focus on thinking, feelings, and behaviors, and grabbing hold of it at the thinking phase, understanding how that contributes to their cycle of relapse." Another stated:

> we tend to get beneath the addiction into how a person thinks and believes; try to deal with people on the soul level with the mind the will and emotions so we look at those things. It may look more therapeutic in our approach than what you may see at a [different program] or a [different program], but it is centered on scripture but with an individual emphasis with the mentors.

From a psychological stance, this is clearly cognitive work, though linguistics often differ between psychological theory and ministry. Another center uses "behavioral modification as a temporary solution to getting behavioral change so we can deal with root problem so then we can deal with it from a spiritual level." One director reiterates that their weakness is a lack of mental health training. Such openness to counseling skills training placed this ministry in the blended category of faith and mental health treatment.

Some use multiple models of treatment approaches. One describes treatment as, "Unique, no one model... Biblically-based but on top of that foundation, I will teach every model possible of addiction recovery available, as long as it doesn't contradict what the Bible says," and they use "12-steps from a Biblical perspective, Rational Recovery, and Rational Emotive Therapy, which is the basis of Rational Recovery...and cognitive-behavioral stuff." Another states they have drawn from "the director's past experience and different models, including [organization] concepts and ideas, Christian psychology concepts, 12-step concepts." They "try to cover all topical areas that are effective in recovery (e.g., codependency), as well as providing basic rudiments of Christian education."

In borrowing aspects of treatment from psychology, these programs remain open to the contribution of biological factors in the etiology and treatment of substance abuse, and allow participants to use psychotropic medication if needed (something that some faith-based programs are opposed to).

Focus on the person in context. This type of care focuses not only on substance abuse, nor solely upon building a relationship with God apart from other aspects of a client's life, but on the real needs present in all areas of life. These may include physical (i.e. housing, food, etc.), educational, vocational, interpersonal, self-efficacy, and recreational needs, while in treatment and afterwards. Several worked hard to provide ample support as clients transition back into the community.

CONCLUSION

These studies demonstrate both the relevance and variance in faith-based substance abuse treatment approaches. The programs that are most useful for church-psychology collaboration are both explicit with a Christian approach to care and also open to incorporating principles from psychology that are used in traditional mental health treatment.

Developing a relationship between treatment-focused ministries and psychological principles seems not only wise from a treatment perspective, but also timely, with the growing interest in church-psychology collaboration (McMinn and Dominguez, 2004). This is one way that an integration of psychology and Christianity can be done on a pragmatic, applicable level. Creating partnerships that incorporate key components of beneficial approaches from the two domains can be done to support a broadened and responsible approach to client care.

REFERENCES

Crits-Christoph, P., Chambless, D. L., Frank, E., Brody, D. and Karp, J. F. (1995). Training in empirically-validated treatments: What are clinical psychology students learning? *Professional Psychology: Research and Practice, 26,* 514-522.

Dominguez, A. D., McMinn, M. R., Lee, T. W., Luka, M., and Steiner-Pappalardo, N. L. (June, 2003). *Substance abuse and the Church: Needs and resources.* Paper presented at the annual meeting of the Christian Association for Psychological Studies. Anaheim, CA.

Garfield, S. L. (1996). Some problems associated with "validated" forms of psychotherapy. *Clinical Psychology, 3,* 218-229.

Greenberg, J. (1994). Psychotherapy research: A clinician's view. In P. F. Talley, H. H. Strupp, and S. F. Butler (Eds.), *Psychotherapy research and practice* (pp. 1-18). New York: Basic Books.

Havik, O. E., and VandenBos, G. R. (1996). Limitations of manualized psychotherapy for everyday clinical practice. *Clinical Psychology, 3,* 264-267.

Hill, P. C., and Pargament, K. I. (2003). Advances in the conceptualization and measurement of religion and spirituality: Implications for physical and mental health research. *American Psychologist, 58.* 64-74.

Lee, T. W., Luka, M., McMinn, M. R., Dominguez, A. W., and Steiner-Pappalardo, N. L. (2004). *Religion and spirituality: Possible confounding factors in substance abuse treatment.* Manuscript submitted for publication.

McMinn, M. R. and Dominguez, A. W. (2004). Psychology and the Church. *Journal of Psychology and Christianity, 22.* 291-292.

Miller, W. R. (1999) (Ed.). *Integrating spirituality into treatment.* Washington, DC: American Psychological Association.

Miller, W. R. and Thoresen, C. E. (2003). Spirituality, religion, and health: An emerging research field. *American Psychologist, 58.* 24-35.

Norcross, J. C. (2002) (Ed.). *Psychotherapy relationships that work.* New York: Oxford University Press.

Powell, L. H., Shahabi, L., and Thoreson, C. E. (2003). Religion and spirituality: Linkages to physical health. *American Psychologist, 58*, 36-52.

Richards, P. S., and Bergin, A. E. (1997). *A spiritual strategy for counseling and psychotherapy.* Washington, DC: American Psychological Association.

Richards, P. S., and Bergin, A. E. (Eds.) (2000). *Handbook of psychotherapy and religious diversity.* Washington, DC: American Psychological Association.

Richards, P. S., and Bergin, A. E. (Eds.) (2004). *Casebook for a spiritual strategy in counseling and psychotherapy.* Washington, DC: American Psychological Association.

Seeman, T. E., Dubin, L. F., and Seeman, M. (2003). Religiosity/spirituality and health: A critical review of the evidence for biological pathways. *American Psychologist, 58*, 54-63.

Shafranske, E. P. (Ed.) (1996a). *Religion and the clinical practice of psychology.* Washington, DC: American Psychological Association.

Silverman, W. H. (1996). Cookbooks, manuals, and paint-by-numbers: Psychotherapy in the 90's. *Psychotherapy, 33, 207-215.*

Talley, P. F., Strupp, H. H., and Butler, S. F. (1994) (Eds.), *Psychotherapy research and practice* (pp. 1-18). New York: Basic Books.

In: Religion and Healthcare   ISBN 978-1-61324-256-8
Editors: A.M. Curtis and D.P. Werthel   © 2012 Nova Science Publishers, Inc.

Chapter 4

SPIRITUAL COPING AMONG CHRONICALLY ILL CHILDREN

Sarah Faith Shelton and Alex P. Mabe

Medical College of Georgia, U.S.A.

ABSTRACT

Children with chronic and potentially life-threatening illnesses are confronted with numerous stressors. Fear and uncertainty regarding the future, unpredictable illness course and outcome, intrusive treatment regimens, invasive medical procedures, perceived or actual loss of control, and general disruption of life events are a few of the many challenges they must face. Numerous studies conducted with chronically ill children support the idea of tailoring treatment to the individual needs of the patient by assessing developmental, familial, and cultural influences. Yet, surprisingly there has been relatively little attention paid in research to the manner in which children use religion/spirituality to help them through these stresses of chronic illness. Adult studies have clearly indicated that many people report turning to their faith beliefs when faced with a crisis such as an illness or an injury. While research on religious/spiritual coping in adults is enjoying growing interest, religious/spiritual coping in children has largely been neglected.

This chapter will review and discuss existing theories and research on children's spiritual coping, specifically as it pertains to dealing with chronic childhood illness. Clinical implications in the field of pediatric psychology and directions for future research in this area will also be explored.

INTRODUCTION

In recent decades there has been a growing interest in the relationship between spirituality and emotional and physical health. Though somewhat limited in number and methodological rigor, there is a growing body of literature that emphasizes that adults are often concerned with spirituality in contexts of suffering, debilitation, and dying. In the United States, religious/spiritual coping appears to be one of the most frequent methods of coping used in response to health-related stressors (Eisenberg et al., 1998, Gall et al., 2005). Roughly 80% of Americans believe that faith through prayer can facilitate healing for themselves and others (Cherry, 1999; Pendleton, Cavalli, Pargament, and Nasr, 2002). In addition, more than half report believing that God has healed them or aided their recovery in the past (Pendleton et al., 2002). In a study of cardiac surgery patients Ai et al. (1998) found that 67.5% of patients reported that private prayer was the most frequently used practice out of a list of 21 non-medical help-seeking or coping behaviors. Other types of religious coping referred to by patients in this study included service attendance (54%), participation in church activities (52%), having faith in God (73%), and praying for guidance following surgery (68%). There is also accumulating evidence in adult health care contexts of a positive association between religion/spirituality and positive health outcomes (George et al., 2000; Levin, 1994; McCullough et al., 2000). The mechanisms by which religion/spirituality might provide health benefits continues to be debated with such factors as increased emotional and social support, expanded psychological resources, and positive health practices as commonly proposed factors.

While attention has increasingly been directed toward the intersection of religion/ spirituality and health, the preponderance of studies have focused on adult participants. This relative neglect of the impact of spirituality on emotional and physical health in children of course does not denote that spirituality has in any less importance for pediatric populations. Also, while it has often been assumed that children utilize their spiritual beliefs to cope with stresses in a manner similar to that of adults, recent findings suggest that this assumption may be at least partially incorrect (Pendleton et al., 2002; Shelton, Linfield, Carter, and Morton, 2005). Thus, conclusions regarding to what extent and how children use spiritual beliefs and practices to cope with health care problems cannot be readily derived from adult spiritual coping studies.

The focus of this article is to examine the nature and impact of spiritual coping on children dealing with the stresses of chronic and potentially life-threatening illnesses. We will focus on the work of Pendleton et al. (2002) and Shelton et al. (2005), as these studies of children with cystic fibrosis and severe asthma effectively illustrate how spirituality may play a vital role in many children's efforts to cope with the stresses of chronic illness. It is proposed that if we are to design effective treatment approaches for children with chronic illness we must better understand how children use their spiritual beliefs and practices in dealing with the stresses of their illnesses.

DEFINING THE CONSTRUCTS

Studying spiritual coping in general has been hindered by the vagaries of the constructs used in this field. Religion and spirituality entail complex and diverse constructs. Religious terms encompass such components as cognition (attributions, beliefs, knowledge), emotion (joy, hope, shame), behavior (church attendance, rituals, prayers, moral actions), and community affiliation (group interactions) (Holden, 2001). Pargament (1990) made the distinction between general measures of religiosity (e.g., church attendance and self-reported importance of religion) and measures of religious coping that could include specific religious practices of prayer, confessing one's sins, and seeking strength and comfort from God in response to a particular stressor. *Religious* has been differentiated from *spiritual*, in that the latter denotes more of the idea of believing in, valuing, or devoting oneself to some higher power without necessarily holding religious beliefs to be true (Worthington et al., 1996). Whereas being religious could involve an individual holding to certain doctrines and practices within a religious organization without necessarily experiencing or expressing any devotion to a higher power other than intellectual assent to its existence.

Given the complexity and diversity of these constructs, it is not surprising that studies involving religion and spirituality often represent diverse psychosocial variables and outcomes. Barnes et al. (2000) pointed out that while people often draw distinctions between religion and spirituality, children generally do not make such distinctions. Fowler (1981) asserted that the constructs of spirituality and religion can become more complex because the child's spiritual beliefs and understanding generally change as the child's cognitive development becomes more advanced and complex. Therefore, it has generally been recommended that in connection with children the constructs of religion and spirituality are best understood as highly related terms with blurred boundaries.

OVERVIEW OF SPIRITUALITY AND HEALTH

The vast majority of studies that have examined the relationship of spirituality and health have not involved children, and it is not clear to what extent these adult studies are relevant for understanding the relationship between spirituality and health in children. Nevertheless, a brief review of general research findings regarding the relationship of spirituality and health seems warranted in order to provide an understanding of how this field of inquiry has evolved.

The nature of research on spirituality as it applies to health began with examining the effects of intercessory prayer. One of the most well known studies of this nature was conducted by Byrd (1988) who evaluated the effects of prayer on coronary patients at San Francisco General Hospital. He found that those who were prayed for were five times less likely to need antibiotics and three times less likely to develop pulmonary edema. In addition, the prayed-for group experienced fewer cases of pneumonia and cardiopulmonary arrest, and fewer patients in this group died compared to the control group. Though controversial, his work is credited with stimulating new interest in the scientific examination of spiritual constructs. Other studies since Byrd's (1988) work have shown that individuals who utilize spiritual resources are at significantly lower risk for development of coronary disease and exhibit lower mortality in the event of diagnosis (George et al., 2000).

A second wave of research on spirituality and health focused on the correlations between spiritual behaviors and positive health factors. For example, regular church attendance has been associated with better immune system functioning, fewer hospital admissions, and shorter hospital stays among elderly individuals (Cherry, 1999). A positive relationship between church attendance and longevity has also been demonstrated, with regular church attendees living an average of 28% longer than those who did not regularly attend church. This statistic parallels the longevity ratio of nonsmokers to smokers (Cherry, 1999; George et al., 2000). Finally, engaging in religious practices (church attendance, prayer, Bible study, etc.) as well as importance placed on spirituality have been found to be associated with lower levels of blood pressure in several studies (Ellison and Smith, 1991; George et al., 2000; Mitka, 1998; Steffen, Hinderliter, Blumenthal, and Sherwood, 2001).

On the whole, more than three-quarters of studies with adults have demonstrated a positive relationship between spirituality and physical health (Cherry, 1999), and very few studies have found spirituality to have a harmful effect on health (George et al., 2000). The exceptions are those religions that have prohibitions against medical interventions in extreme cases, and cults whose rituals involve forms of child abuse (Paloutzian and Kirkpatrick, 1995). Reviews of more than 200 medical studies have concluded that religion/spirituality has a positive influence on health and disease, and that a lack of spirituality is actually a risk factor for illness (Cherry; 1999; George et al., 2000).

Research has also examined how spirituality affects *coping* with physical illness rather than affecting the illness directly. It is this link between spirituality and health that is most pertinent to the work being done in child spiritual coping today. Past research with adult women in various stages of uterine and ovarian cancer credited spirituality with helping them sustain hope in the face of sickness. Edward Creagan, M.D of the Division of Medical Oncology at the Mayo Clinic has noted "among the coping methods of long-term cancer survivors, the predominant (coping) strategy is spiritual" (Ziegler, 1998, 15). Oncology patients who value their spirituality report less subjective pain (frequency and intensity) when compared to non-spiritual oncology patients (Ellison and Smith, 1991). Other studies have demonstrated reduced mortality among breast cancer patients who describe themselves as spiritual (George et al., 2000).

In summary, adult studies have demonstrated that spirituality plays an important role in a broad range of illness related issues, including development, course, outcome, perceptions, and survival of illness. Spirituality also affects patients' coping with illness through means such as decreasing depression and anxiety while increasing hope, pain tolerance, quality of life, and influencing perceptions of one's own health, energy, and vitality (Ellison and Smith, 1991; George et al., 2002). The link between spirituality and health has tended to emphasize the following three main mechanisms:

1) *General Health Behaviors*: Spiritual people are less likely to engage in behaviors that are considered "high risk" with regard to health issues. For instance, some denominations have strict prohibitions against the use of certain chemicals (i.e. alcohol, tobacco), violence, and risky sexual behaviors. Many religious groups view the body as having holy significance and engage in healthy behaviors out of respect for the body's sacred value. While differences can and do exist between and within denominations with regard to these general health behaviors, generally people who view themselves as spiritual

tend to live healthier lifestyles compared to non-spiritual people (George et al., 2000; Paloutzian and Kirkpatrick, 1995).

2) *Social support:* Involvement with a religious institution provides more opportunities for forming close relationships and thus social support. These relationships are likely to lend support, both emotional and instrumental in times of need. Therefore, it is believed that spirituality functions to bolster coping resources and thereby reduce the impact of stress on health and likewise ameliorate the negative effects of illness. The notion that social support is the most potent mechanism of spiritual coping has been widely postulated. However, George et al. (2000) reported that social support accounts for merely 5%-10% of the relationship between health and emotional well being where spirituality is concerned.

3) *Meaning:* Spirituality can provide a sense of meaning and coherence to life events. Believing that events in life have special significance and meaning empowers people with courage and hope thus reducing subjective suffering (Paloutzian and Kirkpatrick, 1995; Paloutzian, and Ellison, 1982). This mechanism has received the most support, accounting for perhaps 20%-30% of the relationship between health and emotional well-being and spirituality (George et al., 2000).

Before concluding this brief listing of the links between spirituality and health, we would be remiss not to mention divine intervention. Bergin and Payne (1993) have pointed out that a person's sense of the supernatural can certainly provide a psychological boost but may also entail a "spiritual boost" that cannot be measured phenomenologically. Although traditionally not considered in scientific contexts because of the transcendental nature of spiritual experience, people of religious faith consistently relate to an understanding of their life experience that entails divine interventions that can change life events, change human thought and behavior, positively influence how one copes with adverse events, and directly impact the state of one's health. Thus although science lends itself better to the study of the psychosocial effects of their spirituality, there is no logical basis to ignore the possibility that spiritual experiences exist that have direct effects on health.

Spiritual Coping

The focus of this article is on spiritual coping, and so it is important to delineate the manner in which this construct has been defined. Spiritual coping consists of unique properties that are not shared by secular coping and is a form or expression of general religion/spirituality. Spiritual coping differs from other spiritual/religious constructs, such as religiosity and religious orientation that are sometimes measured and researched. In fact, measures of spiritual coping more accurately predict the outcomes of negative events than other spiritual/religious measures (Paloutzian and Ellison, 1991). Pendleton et al. (2002, p.1) defined spiritual coping as "a search for significance in times of stress in ways related to the sacred." Religious/spiritual coping has also been defined as entailing cognitive or behavioral techniques that arise out of one's religion or spirituality and are used to address stressful life events (Tix and Frazier, 1998). Pendleton et al. (2002) described spiritual coping as a multidimensional construct, and in adults at least has been implicated in the construction of events, coping processes, and the outcomes pursued. They identified at least 21 religious/spiritual coping strategies in adults that included such efforts as seeking spiritual support that achieves coping via searching for comfort and reassurance through God's love and care. Seeking spiritual support is exemplified by such statements as, "I looked to God for strength, support, and guidance."

Another strategy that Pendleton et al. (2002) described entailed a cognitive reappraisal of their situation from a spiritual perspective. Cognitive reappraisal is exemplified by finding aspects of a negative event that can be considered "blessings in disguise." For example, someone who is unable to work due to illness may focus on the value of spending more time at home with family as opposed to focusing on the loss of things associated with a former job, such as income and work-related productivity and identity. In summary, definitions of spiritual coping have generally pointed to a reliance on one's spiritual's beliefs or practices in an attempt to influence positive change in a situation or in one's ability to deal with a situation.

Spirituality and the Chronically Ill Child

Children facing chronic and potentially life-threatening illness are certainly faced with numerous stressors (Albano, Causey, and Carter, 2000; Forman, 1993). Fear, anger, separation from home and environment, and perceived or actual lack of control are among the problems with which these children must cope. Chronic illness often represents a state of uncertainty, manifested primarily by unfamiliar and novel experiences, the unpredictable nature of the illness trajectory, and uncertain outcomes. In addition, the chronically ill child is often confronted with physical pain and discomfort, concerns about body integrity, and invasive medical procedures (Kronenberger, Carter, and Thomas, 1997). Moreover, the demands faced by children with chronic illness affect multiple life domains, including biological changes, management of regimens, social stressors, and disruptions in normal routines and activities (Amer, 1999). The most commonly cited stressor for children with chronic illness has been the intrusiveness of the illness into everyday life, particularly illness symptoms and the rigor of illness-management regimens that require medications and/or treatments, self-care skills, and constant monitoring for reactions and side effects. Stewart (2003) reported that in addition to their toll on children's physical and emotional stamina, the demands of chronic illness and their associated treatment regimens reverberate into two important areas of children's lives: (1) they constrain children's participation in normal everyday activities such as sports, recreation, and school and (2) as a result of the visibility of self care regimens, such as taking medications or monitoring blood glucose levels during the school day, they amplify differences with their peers.

Studies of how children cope with chronic illness have commonly cited their seeking social support as a primary coping strategy. Children often seek out support from family, peers, and professionals in dealing with the multiple stresses and demands of chronic illness. This social support takes the form of affirmation, emotional comfort and presence during difficult times, information, and distraction from illness concerns (Stewart, 2003). Amer (1999) reported that some children developed "compensatory attributes," personal interests and abilities that offset physical or social deficits imposed by chronic illness.

Another interesting strategy commonly observed among children coping with chronic illness has been the use of repression (Phipps and Steele, 2002). Studies of children with a variety of chronic illnesses suggest that many of these children often under-report emotional distress, and this repressive adaptation can occur as both an acutely reactive phenomena and a style of long-term adaptation. A perplexing issue, however, is the question of whether repression in the context of serious illness is adaptive. Certainly, in the face of highly threatening circumstances such as the onset of a catastrophic illness, the ability to block out or limit awareness of anxiety-provoking stimuli could be beneficial. On the other hand, this repressive adaptation could lead to a reluctance to seek social support and a lack of attention to internal signals of distress, including physical symptoms that could delay effective medical intervention.

Surprisingly, very few studies have examined if and in what way children use spirituality to help them through these periods of crisis. The small pool of published research on children's spiritual coping primarily addresses spirituality in the context of health behaviors such as substance abuse and sexual activity, trauma, and bereavement processes (e.g. Barnes et al., 2000; Nierenberg and Sheldon, 2001). The authors of this chapter conducted an extensive literature review using six major journal databases that generated articles related to psychology, medicine, nursing, and education over the past decade or more and discovered only two published studies (Pendleton et al., 2002; Shelton et al., 2005) that directly examine child spiritual coping in relation to illness. Other articles touch on the need for spiritual assessment and integration into pediatric treatment, but most of these are rationally driven with little or no empirical evidence to support what seem to be very logical assertions (e.g. Elkins and Cavendish, 2004). Overall there appears to be striking absence of theological contributions in the research of coping with health and wellness concerns among pediatric populations.

Spiritual Coping in Children with Pulmonary Disorders

The two studies of spiritual coping in children that we will review involve children with pulmonary disorders of cystic fibrosis (CF) and/or asthma. CF is the most common inherited disease among Caucasians with a fatal outcome in industrialized nations and is becoming increasingly prevalent as survival is prolonged. With improved treatment regimens, the life expectancy of children with CF has increased from 7.5 years in 1966 to a median of 31.3 years for men and 28.3 years for women in the United States in 1999 (Jackson and Vessey, 2000). Despite advances in understanding the genetics and pathophysiology of CF, a curative treatment remains elusive. Thus children with CF continue to have to endure complex and time consuming therapeutic regimens consisting of chest physiotherapy, inhalation therapy, pancreatic enzyme supplements, and regular antibiotic treatments with an uncertain life expectancy outcome. Children with CF also experience recurrent illness-related events such as pain, repeated medical procedures, fear of death, and the embarrassment of being physically different from other children (Thompson and Gustafson, 1996).

Asthma is currently the most common childhood chronic illness and affects more than 6% of children in the United States (NHLBI, 1999). Despite advances in the understanding of the pathogenesis of asthma and improvements in treatment approaches, national statistics reveal increasing morbidity and mortality from asthma in the past decade. Children with severe asthma experience recurrent and unpredictable apnea events that can be quite frightening and disruptive to their life functioning and, like children with CF, they must engage in daily routines of pulmonary/inhalant therapy. The morbidity of asthma is considerable for children being one of the leading causes of lost days in school, physician contacts, and hospitalizations (Taylor and Newacheck, 1992).

The conditions of CF and severe asthma certainly represent formidable adaptation challenges for children. Therefore, efforts to understand how children might attempt to cope with the stresses inherent in these illnesses would be informative with regard to the field of spiritual coping in children as well as the broader field of children coping with chronic illness. We will now review two studies that have examined the spiritual coping of children with CF or severe asthma.

Pendleton et al. (2002)

Pendleton et al. (2002) conducted an exploratory study to examine the spiritual coping of children with CF. Participants consisted of 23 patients, ranging in age from 5 to 12 years of age, who attended an out-patient CF clinic. The religious demographics of participants in this study reflected the national distribution with 48% Protestant, 26% Catholic, 4% Jewish, 4% Native American religion, 4% classified as Other, and 9% with no religious affiliation. All participants in this study were Caucasian (which reflects the genetic predisposition of cystic fibrosis). In-depth open-ended interviews with the children were the primary means of investigation. Children were also asked to draw themselves and God when they are sick and to explain their drawings as part of the interview process. Parental questionnaires assessing the importance of spirituality in themselves and their children were also evaluated. Six hundred and thirty-two quotes gleaned from the interviews were coded. Grounded theory analysis produced one overarching domain of spiritual coping along with 11 themes or strategies. They were as follows (Pendleton et al., 2002, 7):

1. "Declarative Religious/Spiritual Coping" which consists of the child making a statement about what will happen and expecting God to do it automatically. When using this strategy, children expressed the unchallenged belief that God will act on their requests while denying the possibility that God may not honor their requests for various reasons.

2. "Petitionary Religious/Spiritual Coping" which is demonstrated by the child appealing to God and believing that there is a possibility (rather than an absolute certainty) of influencing outcomes via their request. Unlike declarative religious/spiritual coping, this strategy allows for factors, such as nature, that could explain how or why their requests may not be honored. No children, however, reported believing that God does not want to help them.

3. "Collaborative Religious/Spiritual Coping" which represents the perspective that the child and God work together as a team. This strategy assumes that both God and the child play a somewhat equal role in the outcome.

4. "Belief in God's Support" which represents the child's general belief that God will help, benefit, and comfort him or her. For example, use of this strategy consists of the child believing that God will provide or assist in the development of qualities such as courage, which will not necessarily affect the situation, but will enhance the child's ability to endure the situation.

5. "Belief in God's Intervention" which is exemplified by the child's belief that God intervenes to affect the stressor in a divine and supernatural way. Unlike declarative religious/spiritual coping, God may act without the child's request or command. This strategy also differs from belief in God's support, because in "Belief in God's Intervention," God addresses the stressor as opposed to the child.

6. "Belief that God is Irrelevant" which occurs when the child does not rely on God because he or she either has no knowledge of God, does not believe God is important, or believes that God is uninvolved. Not surprisingly, this strategy played a bigger role among children with limited beliefs or limited exposure to religion/spirituality.

7. "Spiritual Social Support" which consists of the child, other people, and God interacting to provide guidance, comfort, and support. This

can take the form of group or mutual prayer, group identity and activities, and practical support such as food and clothing provided by individuals from the child's religious/spiritual community.

8. "Ritual Response" which consists of the child engaging in activities with religious symbolic significance in order to influence stressors (e.g., church attendance or prayer). Few children in this study reported relying on this strategy.

9. "Benevolent Religious/Spiritual Reappraisal" which occurs when the child reframes the situation or God's response in a positive manner. This may take the form of placing religious/spiritual meaning on the stressor. For example, a child might believe that he/she is experiencing sickness first-hand as a child, so that he/she can grow up to become a good pediatrician as an adult. The child may also make an undesired response by God seem less negative by placing limitations on God's power. This tactic was strongly preferred over entertaining the notion that God denied their request. Interestingly, no child made reference to God's will as a reason for undesired outcomes.

10. "Punishing Religious/Spiritual Reappraisal" which occurs when the child perceives the stressor as a punishment from God. No child reported that his or her stressor was directly punishment, but some believed punishment could occur.

11. "Discontent with God or Congregation" which consists of the child expressing disappointment in or anger at God and/or people, such as fellow church members, associated with God. Children were more likely to report feeling disappointed as opposed to angry.

Comparing their findings in this child study to models of religious/spiritual coping developed and tested in adults, Pendleton et al. (2002) noted the following main differences between spiritual coping in children versus adults: First, adults do not exhibit a declarative spiritual strategy as do children. Second, children are significantly less likely to endorse negative forms of spiritual coping, such as punishing reappraisal or discontent, compared to adults. Third, children's spiritual coping strategies are generally less sophisticated than adults. Adults' spiritual coping strategies are differentiated by subtleties, whereas children's spiritual coping strategies are differentiated by starker contrasts. For example, adults seem to distinguish between prayer by others on their behalf, prayer from a religious authority (such as a priest, rabbi, or minister), and prayers generated by the self.

Children, on the other hand, seem to view all prayer as equally desirable, beneficial, and effective.

The analyses of this qualitative study highlighted the overarching importance of spiritual coping in children's efforts to cope with CF, as most of the children in their sample associated their individual religiousness/ spirituality with coping. Moreover, their results pointed to the multidimensional nature of spiritual coping, as their typology identified at least 11 strategies with spiritual meanings. Finally, this study magnified the importance of addressing the patient's and family's belief system in health related treatment.

Shelton et al. (2005)

While Pendleton et al.'s study (2002) added light to our understanding of the extent and nature of spiritual coping in children coping with CF, it did not assess the impact of these coping efforts on emotional and behavior disturbance that are common among children with severe asthma and CF. Also, Pendleton et al.'s (2002) study identified spiritual coping strategies that were rationally as opposed to empirically derived. While a good start in attempting to understand spiritual coping among children, this method of identifying spiritual coping strategies is less desirable than more objective efforts such as statistical analysis.

Building on Pendleton et al.'s study (2002) of spiritual coping in children with CF, Shelton et al. (2005) investigated if and in what manner spiritual coping mediated emotional and behavioral disturbances among children with CF or severe asthma. Children with CF and severe asthma were chosen for study because both illness conditions represented chronic and life-threatening illnesses that imposed significant stresses on children as a result of their unpredictable symptoms and illness course, and their high maintenance medical regimens. In fact, studies of children with CF have generally concluded that they are particularly at increased risk for anxiety and oppositional disorders (e.g., Thompson et al., 1998). Likewise, children with severe asthma also have been found to be vulnerable for emotional and behavioral disturbances. Although unlike children with CF, children with asthma appear to exhibit more problems with anxiety and depression rather than oppositional or hyperactive behavior problems (McQuaid, Kopel, and Nassau, 2001). Study of these chronic illness conditions thus afforded the opportunity to examine to what extent spiritual coping might influence their stress related symptoms. In addition, conducting research with children with CF and asthma provided a degree of continuity with Pendleton et al.'s (2002) earlier work on spiritual coping among pediatric pulmonary patients.

Shelton et al. (2005) examined to what extent spiritual coping reduces the tendency for pediatric pulmonary patients to react adversely (behaviorally and emotionally) to their medical situation. Also of interest in this study was the relationship between spiritual coping in pediatric pulmonary patients and their overall adjustment to illness as denoted by compliance with medical procedures and degree of impairment/interruption to life (missed school days and number of emergency room visits and hospitalizations due to diagnosis). Finally, Shelton et al. (2005) set out to identify spiritual coping strategies by empirical as opposed to rational methods, in order to improve on the research methodology in this area.

Participants consisted of 100 parent-child sets, in which the child was a patient of a pediatric pulmonary clinic affiliated with a children's hospital in the southeast United States. Child participants had diagnoses of cystic fibrosis or level 3 (moderate persistent) to level 4 (severe) asthma. Ages of the children ranged from 6 years to 16 years of age, with a mean age of 11 years. There were 49 males, 50 females, and 1 child whose parent declined to indicate gender on a demographic questionnaire. There were 62 Caucasians, 21 African-Americans, 3 Hispanics, 2 Native Americans, 5 whose parents endorsed "Other," and 7 children whose parents declined to indicate race on a demographic questionnaire. Religious denominations of the participants consisted of 83 children of Christian faith, 3 children of Jewish faith, 1 child whose parent specified "Other" on a demographic questionnaire, 5 Agnostics, and 3 Atheists.

Parents of all child participants were administered a demographic questionnaire and the Spiritual Well-Being Scale (SWB; Paloutzian and Ellison, 1991) that provided a global measure of the parents' subjective quality of life. The Behavior Assessment System for Children (BASC; Reynolds and Kamphaus, 1992) provided ratings of child emotional and behavioral disturbances. The BASC Parent Rating Scales produces composite indices of Externalizing Problems (e.g., aggression, hyperactivity, and conduct problems), Internalizing Problems (e.g., depression, anxiety, and somatization), and a Behavioral Symptoms Index (i.e., a composite of externalizing and internalizing symptoms). The BASC Self-Report produces an Emotional Symptoms Index, which represents primarily problems with mood, relationships with others, and a sense of one's personal adjustment. For children under the age of 12, the Parent Rating Scales of the BASC were obtained, whereas for children 12 years and older the Self-Report of the BASC was obtained. Children's overall adjustment to illness was assessed by items on the demographic questionnaire completed by parents and provided indices of the number of emergency room visits, hospitalizations, and missed school days due to diagnosis in the12-month period prior to participating in the study. Compliance with medical treatment was also obtained on the demographic questionnaire and entailed the parent's rating of the child's compliance on a 5-point scale.

Shelton et al. (2005) rationally derived items to reflect eight of the eleven spiritual coping strategies found in Pendleton et al.'s (2002) sample. Ten items were created for each of the eight spiritual coping strategies selected for a total of 80 preliminary items. This list of preliminary items was given to 18 students and graduates of various Protestant seminaries in order to establish content validity of the spiritual coping items. Seminary students were asked to rate each item in terms of how strongly it represented the concept it was meant to embody using a 5-point rating scale ranging from 1 = "definitely does" to 5 = "definitely does not" capture the concept. After analyzing the results, 24 items (the three best rated items for each of the eight domains) were selected from the original 80 sample items in order to develop a more concise and valid measure to be administered to children. All child participants completed this 24-item measure of children's spiritual coping that yielded a global spiritual coping index and, as described below, produced four distinct spiritual coping strategies as well.

Key findings for the global spiritual coping index revealed that children who engaged in higher levels of spiritual coping tended to report lower levels of general emotional distress (i.e., lower scores on the Emotional Symptoms Index of the BASC Self Report) as obtained from children 12 years of age and older. In contrast, children's spiritual coping was not associated with lower levels of a global composite of internalizing and externalizing behavioral problems (i.e., the Behavioral Symptoms Index on the BASC Parent Rating Scales) as obtained from the parents of children younger that 12 years of age. Due to the correlational design employed and the variation of measures used based on the age of the child, it is difficult to discern the precise nature of these discrepant findings. Nevertheless, we would propose the hypothesis that the discrepant findings lend themselves to the interpretation that global spiritual coping may provide benefits for children in dealing with their internal states of distress more so than for the management of their externalizing-behavioral problems. The logic of this hypothesis follows from previous child-parent rating comparisons that have noted that parents have been shown to be reasonably good raters of externalizing behaviors (e.g., aggression, hyperactivity, conduct problems) in their children but relatively poor raters of internalizing symptoms (e.g., anxiety, depression, somatization) (Weiner et al., 1987; Yule, 1993); whereas children tend to be more able in providing assessment of their own internal states than outside observers (i.e., parents, teachers, or peers). Consequently, if spiritual coping provides the most benefit for reducing internal distress, then it would not be surprising that the BASC Self Report Emotional Symptoms Index was correlated with spiritual coping while the BASC Parent Rating Scales did not yield significant correlations with spiritual coping.

With regard to response to treatment and overall adjustment to illness variables, children who engaged in higher levels of spiritual coping tended to have fewer emergency room visits due to their diagnosis. However, no significant relationships were found between children's overall level of spiritual coping and compliance with medical treatment, number of missed school days due to diagnosis, or number of hospitalizations due to diagnosis. Again, the nature of these discrepant findings is difficult to discern from this study, but we would we continue to emphasize the link between spiritual coping and internal states of distress as a possible explanatory factor. More specifically, we would propose that emergency room visits for children with pulmonary disease are more likely to be influenced by their internal states of distress than would be the case for the other illness adjustment indices (i.e., regimen compliance, hospitalizations, and missed school days). Difficulties with breathing that are interpreted by children and adults as requiring urgent care can be readily influenced by internal states of distress more so than decisions involving such matters as hospitalization in which objective medical findings after a period of careful evaluation are more likely to come into play. Thus if spiritual coping reduces internal states of distress in children then it would predictably have a benefit in reducing the same distress factors that could adversely influence breathing or the interpretation of breathing problems – both factors that can trigger emergency room visits.

In regard to social/demographic correlates of global spiritual coping in children the findings were logically quite predictable. Children who embraced a particular faith (e.g. Jewish, Christian) tended to have higher levels of global spiritual coping compared to children who did not embrace a particular faith (e.g. Agnostic, Atheist). Also, children with higher levels of spiritual coping tended to have parents with higher levels of global spiritual well-being (as measured by the SWB Scale). Thus as would be expected children with more opportunities to observe and be taught spiritual/religious beliefs and practices are more likely to use spiritual coping than those children with limited exposure to others practicing their faith.

Further Delineating the Nature of Children's Spiritual Coping

As previously described, Shelton et al. (2005) devised and administered a measure of spiritual coping for chronically ill children based on eight of the eleven strategies delineated by Pendleton et al. (2002). Using varimax rotation with Kaiser normalization, of the eight domains of spiritual coping specified and included on the children's spiritual coping measure only four strategies of children's spiritual coping were gleaned. The four spiritual coping strategies that emerged from the factor analysis of Shelton et al.'s (2005) research were: Declarative Spiritual Coping, Petitionary Spiritual Coping, Intervening Spiritual Coping, and Faith Spiritual Coping. Both the Declarative Spiritual Coping strategy (the child commands God to do something and expects God to oblige with no possibility of the command not being followed) and the Petitionary Spiritual Coping strategy (the child believes that asking God to intervene may increase the likelihood of God acting on his/her behalf, but the possibility exists for the request to not result in change) were similar to Pendleton et al.'s (2002) description of those strategies. Based on the results of the factor analysis, Shelton et al. (2005) proposed a third strategy they termed Intervening Spiritual Coping. Most of the items that loaded onto this factor had in common a general sense that God is benevolent and is going to intervene in regard to the illness outcome but the child believes that his/her actions do not have a direct role in influencing specific outcomes. In other words for Intervening Spiritual Coping the child does not hold the belief that he/she can direct the manner in which God will intervene. Shelton et al. (2005) also proposed a fourth strategy based on results of the factor analysis they termed Faith Spiritual Coping. The majority of items that loaded onto this factor had in common trusting a higher power within a collaborative relationship and believing in that power's ability to intervene in some way but that outcome may entail either a positive illness outcome or strengthening of the child's ability to cope with the illness outcome through social/emotional resources or finding meaning or purpose in their illness stresses.

Consistent with the global spiritual coping findings, all four spiritual coping strategies were negatively corrected with the general emotional distress (i.e., scores on the Emotional Symptoms Index of the BASC Self Report) as obtained from children 12 and older. Apparently, the use of any of the four spiritual coping strategies was associated with better emotional health in children 12 and older. Thus any of the four forms of spiritual coping in combination or in isolation may be advantageous strategies for this population in regard to emotional distress. However, the correlations between Intervening Spiritual Coping and Faith Spiritual Coping with global emotional distress ($r = - 0.47$ and $r = - 0.52$, $p < .01$, respectively) were particularly strong. Perhaps both of these latter spiritual strategies provide a coping advantage for children because they both allow for a broader view of a what constitutes a positive outcome in their illness circumstances and thus are less susceptible to the disappointments of not achieving a specific desired illness outcome. Children who engaged in higher levels of Faith Spiritual Coping also tended to have fewer emergency room visits related to their diagnosis. This finding implies that the use of this strategy may be particularly useful in preventing or quelling panic and anxiety symptoms that may contribute to the perception of or actual occurrence of a medical emergency, especially with regard to breathing patterns.

Shelton et al.'s (2005) study reported differences in degree and style of spiritual coping with regard to demographic variables including age, gender, and faith orientation. There was a significant relationship between age and three of the four spiritual coping factors. Younger children tended to rely more heavily on Declarative Spiritual Coping and Intervening Spiritual Coping, while older children tended to use the strategy of Faith Spiritual Coping more often. The finding that younger children tended to use Declarative Spiritual Coping and Intervening Spiritual Coping is consistent with the generally accepted view that young children are more likely to hold diffuse and generalized impressions of their experiences as well as to employ concrete operations to act on those experiences. Consequently, younger children are more likely to hold the unquestioned belief that God will intervene on their behalf to improve the circumstances of their lives whether God is specifically directed by their actions or not. Older children, on the other hand, appear to hold more complex views of God's actions in their lives in that while they maintain a broad sense of God's benevolence they understand that help may come in many different forms that may or may not involve improvement in the circumstances of their lives.

Gender differences were also found with regard to use of specific spiritual coping strategies. Females tended to engage in Intervening Spiritual Coping and Faith Spiritual Coping to a greater degree than males, while males tended to engage in Petitionary Spiritual Coping more so than females. Declarative Spiritual Coping was not shown to be related to gender in any way, which is not surprising given that this strategy is utilized most by younger children whose gender differences are not as pronounced.

There were also significant relationships between spiritual orientation and three of the four coping strategies investigated. Children who embraced a particular faith system tended to engage in Petitionary Spiritual Coping, Intervening Spiritual Coping, and Faith Spiritual Coping more so than children who did not adopt a particular faith system. We would propose that children with greater exposure to a faith system and spiritual activities of others are more likely to be socialized to engage in spiritual strategies with more "flexibility" in how God is viewed as helping them.

CONCLUSION

As presented in this review, our understanding of children's spirituality in the context of coping with chronic illness is very rudimentary. In the context of children with pulmonary disease, both Pendleton et al. (2002) and Shelton et al. (2005) reported that spiritual coping is a common strategy among children dealing with the stresses associated with chronic illnesses. In both Pendleton et al.'s (2002) and Shelton et al.'s (2005) studies, virtually all children endorsed some form of spiritual coping, even among children who classified themselves as atheist. In their efforts to define and refine what the construct of spiritual coping represents for children with chronic illness, we note three fundamental themes.

First, spiritual coping in children appears to be a much less complex and less differentiated construct than with adults. While Pendleton et al. (2002) identified at least 21 spiritual coping strategies in adults, Pendleton et al.'s (2002) study of spiritual coping in children dealing with CF produced one overarching domain of spiritual coping along with only 11 themes or strategies based on their grounded theory analysis.

Using factor analysis, Shelton et al.'s (2005) study of children coping with CF or severe asthma empirically derived only 4 spiritual coping strategies in addition to a broad domain of spiritual coping. The relative immaturity in children's spiritual coping of course parallels their simplistic conceptualizations of life stresses in general and their more limited repertoire of coping strategies. Further study is needed to understand how children move from their relatively immature spiritual coping strategies to the more complex and differentiated spiritual coping strategies observed in adults.

Second, in the examination of Shelton et al.'s (2005) empirically derived strategies there appears to be one dominant theme: children expect God to benevolently intervene in their illness situation. There are variations regarding the extent to which children believe that they direct or participate in God's intervention. Also, there are variations regarding the degree of certainty that they hold regarding God's intervention. Nevertheless, for children there appears to be a consistent sense of God's benevolence, and we would propose that their spiritual coping efforts likely benefit primarily from an expectation that God will somehow change their life circumstances for the better. This emphasis on positive expectations of God's intervention places children's spiritual coping predominately in the category of a cognitive appraisal strategy. That is, spiritual coping for children appears to center more around belief about one's circumstances rather than some behavioral technique or religious practice or association with others of like faith. Given this reliance on a positive expectation for God's intervention, interesting questions arise regarding the nature and effect of children's spiritual coping during the progression of an illness. For example, what happens when illness outcomes are progressively negative? How do children maintain a belief in God's benevolence and how long will this view be maintained in the face of mounting negative outcomes as might be observed with CF? Further longitudinal study of children's spiritual coping is needed along with time analyses of spiritual coping and negative illness outcomes. Children's cognitive appraisal of God's intervention could be considered akin to the repression that has been observed among children with chronic illness. Similar to repression, in the face of highly threatening circumstances spiritual coping may provide the child the ability to block out or limit awareness of anxiety-provoking stimuli. On the other hand, like repression, does spiritual coping lead to a reluctance to seek social support and a lack of attention to internal signals of distress, including physical symptoms, which could delay appropriate medical intervention? This potential adverse effect of spiritual coping is deserving of additional research attention. Future studies of spiritual coping in children need to consider the relationship and impact of spiritual coping on other coping strategies that children and their families use in the context of illness.

Third, Shelton et al.'s (2005) study provided findings that support the view that spiritual coping is influenced by a socialization process. Young children and children not exposed to a faith system were more likely to hold the "naïve view" that they could direct God to intervene in specific ways without any doubt that God would deliver. As children grow older and apparently with more exposure to a faith system, however, they seem more likely to accept the view that they are at best participants in God's interventions in their lives and the specific outcome that they would desire (i.e., better illness outcome) may or may not be achieved. There also seems to be a progression in the complexity of children's thinking about outcomes such that they come to believe that the positive outcome achieved could be their ability to cope with negative outcomes as well as an actual improvement in their illness condition. It should be noted that with few exceptions most mainstream religious faith systems in our country teach a perspective on God that would be more in line with this more developmentally mature perspective on God and divine interventions in their lives. Thus it is likely that as children grow older they become more and more influenced by their faith system and its teachings regarding God's intervention. Of interest would be study of the potential influence of illness events themselves on the development of children's spiritual coping. Perhaps with the exposure to adverse illness outcomes children with chronic illness (and their siblings) develop precociously in their spiritual coping strategies compared with healthy children who have not had their spiritual perspectives so challenged.

The two studies that have examined children's spiritual coping reflect a generally positive view of spirituality as a potentially helpful tool for coping with the stresses inherent in chronic illness. In Pendleton et al.'s (2002) study it was reported that children with CF almost always associated spiritual coping with adaptive health outcomes. Shelton et al.'s (2005) study of children with CF or severe asthma also reported that spiritual coping had positive benefits but the benefits were primarily related to reducing children's emotional distress. It was also noteworthy that the apparent benefits of spiritual coping for children in reducing emotional distress were observed in older children rather than younger children. This later finding of an age influence may have been confounded by a methodological problem with the study in that the self-report of internal distress was only available for children 12 years of age and older, whereas the younger children's internal distress was only measured through parent report. In Shelton et al.'s (2005) study, spiritual coping was not associated with such disease coping outcomes as behavioral or emotional distress symptoms observed by the parents, treatment regimen compliance, hospitalizations, or lost days in school. On the other hand, Shelton et al.'s (2005) findings did suggest a link between spiritual coping and reduction in emergency room visits. We proposed that this reduction in emergency room visits may be linked to the effect of spiritual coping on reducing emotional distresses in children so as to reduce the panic that may precipitously result in a child-family seeking urgent care. Neither study suggested that spiritual coping had an adverse effect on children's emotions, behaviors, or disease outcomes. Perhaps all that can be concluded at this early state of development in the field is that spiritual coping in dealing with chronic illness is viewed favorably by children and their families and for older children appears to reduce their own perceived emotional distress symptoms.

As with most exploratory and correlational studies of a new field, the research implications of these studies would seem to point to an association of spiritual coping and adaptation to chronic illness for children that is worthy of further research. Similar exploratory methodologies need to be applied to other disease contexts that are known to entail significant adaptation challenges (e.g., diseases of the central nervous system, childhood cancer, and diabetes). It is conceivable that other disease conditions may pose different adaptation challenges and thus exhibit different associations with spiritual coping. The methodological limitations of these first two exploratory studies in examining the relationship of spiritual coping and emotional distress symptoms of young children need to be addressed in future studies as well. In particular, efforts need to be made to include self-perceptions of emotional distress symptoms in younger children as part of spiritual coping study.

The clinical implications of this review are necessarily limited given the immature stage of research development in spiritual coping in children. Yet, numerous studies conducted with chronically ill and injured children support the idea of tailoring treatment to the individual needs of the patient by assessing familial, developmental, personality, emotional, and other influences (Albano, Causey, and Carter, 2000; Stearns, Smith, and Carter, 2000). Moreover, research cited in this review suggests that the role that chronically ill children assign spirituality is an important facet of children's coping that should be considered in order to fully understand their experience of chronic illness and to aid in selecting an optimal comprehensive treatment plan. Therefore, we would propose that children's spirituality should be routinely assessed by health care providers in order to ascertain if, and to what degree, children place value on their own spiritual beliefs.

The FICA model of integrating spirituality into the physicians' assessment of patients provides a useful guideline of how to address spirituality with patients of all ages, including children (Puchalski et al., 1999). The patient's developmental level is taken into consideration with regard to depth and focus of the interview. An increasing number of medical schools are teaching the FICA acronym as a technique in courses on spirituality and medicine and entails the following assessment algorithm (Puchalski et al., 1999, 1):

"F- Faith and Beliefs." The physician inquires what, if any, faith is important to the patient. This question should be simple and broad, such as "Are you a religious or spiritual person?"

"I- Importance and Influence." If the answer to the first question is positive, then the physician inquires about the emphasis the individual places on these beliefs.

"C- Community." The physician asks if the patient experiences his or her spiritual life in the context of an identifiable community. This is useful information, in that it indicates the likelihood of social and practical support.

"A- Address and Application." The physician asks the patient if and how he or she would like these beliefs incorporated into the physician-patient relationship. There will be variability across patients with regard to this question. Some patients may ask for a clergy referral, particularly in the event of life-threatening circumstances (Puchalski et al., 1999). Other patients will not wish to discuss their beliefs any further. Yet research has demonstrated that the vast majority of patients appreciate the inquiry of religion/spirituality by healthcare professionals, even among those who decline to integrate their belief system into their healthcare (Allen, 1980).

Of course with children this FICA guideline needs to include the family as part of the assessment. Given the prevalence and potential benefits of spiritual coping in children and their families dealing with chronic illness we believe that it behooves health care professionals to better understand, normalize, and facilitate spiritual coping in children in a manner that respects children's pre-existing spiritual belief system. What lies ahead is a better understanding of how the health care professional as well as families can foster the development of more mature and perhaps more effective spiritual coping strategies in children.

REFERENCES

Ai A.L., Dunkle R.E., Peterson C., Bolling S.F. (1998). The role of private prayer in psychological recovery among midlife and aged patients following cardiac surgery. *Gerontologist*, 38 (5), 591-601.

Albano, A.M., Causey, D., and Carter, B.D. (2000). In C.E. Walker and M.C. Roberts (Eds.), *Handbook of clinical child psychology.* (3rd Ed.) New York: Wiley and Sons, 291-316.

Allen, D., Bird, L., and Herman, R. (1980). The ministry of medicine in the care of the whole person. *Whole-person medicine: An international symposium.* Downer's Grove, IL: InterVarsity Press, 231.

Amer K.S. (1999). Children's adaptation to insulin dependent diabetes mellitus: A critical review of the literature. *Pediatric Nursing,* 25 (6), 627-31, 635-41.

Barnes, L.L., Plotnikoff G.A., Fox K., Pendleton, S. (2000). Spirituality, religion, and pediatrics: Intersecting worlds of healing. *Pediatrics,* 106, 899-908.

Bergin A.E., Payne I.R. (1993). . Proposed agenda for a spiritual strategy in personality and psychotherapy. In E.L Worthington (Ed.) *Psychotherapy and religious values.* Grand Rapids, MI: Baker, 243-260.

Byrd, R. (1988). Positive therapeutic effects of intercessory prayer in a coronary care unit population. *Southern Medical Journal,* 826-829.

Cherry, R. (1999). *Healing prayer.* Nashville, TN: Thomas Nelson Publishers, 3-21.

Eisenberg, D.M., David, R.B., Ettner, S..L, et al. (1998). Trends in alternative medicine use in the United States, 1990-1997: Results of a follow-up national survey. *JAMA* 280, 1569-1575.

Elkins, M. and Cavendish, R. (2004). Developing a plan for pediatric spiritual care. *Holistic Nursing Practice,* 18 (4), 179-184.

Ellison, C.W. (1983). Spiritual well-being: Conceptualization and measurement. *Journal of Psychology and Theology,* 11, 330-340.

Ellison, C.W. and Smith, J. (1991). Toward and integrative measure of health and well-being. *Journal of Psychology and Theology,* 19 (1). 35-48.

Forman, S.G. (1993). *Coping skills interventions for children and adolescents.* San Francisco: Jossey-Bass Publishers, 1-15.

Fowler, J. (1981). Stages of faith: The psychology of human development and the quest for meaning. New York: HarperCollins.

Gall et al. (2005). Understanding the nature and role of spirituality in relation to coping and health: A conceptual framework. *Canadian Psychology,* 46 (2), 88-104.

George L.K., Larson, D.B., Koenig, H.G., McCullough, M.E. (2000). Spirituality and Health: What we know, what we need to know. *Journal of Social and Clinical Psychology,* 19, 102–116.

Holden, G.W. (2001). Psychology, religion, and the family: It's time for a revival. *Journal of Family Psychology,* 15, 657-662.

Jackson, P. L., and Vessey, J. A. (2000). *Child with a chronic condition.* St. Louis, MO: C. V. Mosby.

Kronenberger, W.G., Carter, B.D., and Thomas, D. (1997). Assessment of behavior problems in pediatric inpatient settings: Development of the Pediatric Inpatient Behavior Scale. *Children's Health Care*, 26 (4), 211-232.

Levin, J.S. (1994). Religion and health: Is there an association, is it valid and is it causal? *Social Science of Medicine*, 38, 1475–1482.

McCullough, M.E., Hoyt, W.T., Larson, D.B., Koenig, H.G., and Thoresen, C. (2000). Religious involvement and mortality: A meta-analytic review. *Health Psychology*, 19, 211–222.

McQuaid, E.L., Kopel, S.J., Nassau, J.H. (2001). Behavioral adjustment in children with asthma: A meta-analysis. *Journal of Developmental and Behavioral Pediatrics,* 22 (6), 430-439.

Nierenberg, B. and Sheldon, A. (2001). Psychospirituality and pediatric rehabilitation. *Journal of Rehabilitation,* 67 (1), 15-19.

NHLBI (1999). *Asthma Statistics Data Fact Sheet.* Bethesda, MD, National Heart, Lung, and Blood Institute.

Paloutzian, R.F., and Ellison, C.W. (1982). In L.A. Peplau and D. Perlman (Eds.). *Loneliness: A sourcebook of current theory, research, and therapy.* New York: Wiley-Interscience, 224-237.

Paloutzian, R.F., and Ellison, C.W. (1991). Manual for the Spiritual Well-Being Scale.

Paloutzian, R.F. and Kirkpatrick, L.A. (1995). Introduction: The scope of religious influence on personal and societal well-being. *Journal of Social Issues,* 51 (2), 1-11.

Pargament, K.I. (1990). In M.L. Lynn and D.O. Moberg (Eds.) *God help me: Towards a theoretical framework of coping for the psychology of religion.* Greenwich, CT: JAI Press, 195-224.

Pargament, K.I. (1997). *The psychology of religion and coping: theory, research, practice.* New York: Guilford Press.

Pendleton, S.M., Cavalli, K.S., Pargament, K.I., and Nasr., S.Z. (2002). Religious/spiritual coping in childhood cystic fibrosis: A qualitative study. *Pediatrics,* 109 (1), 1-11.

Phipps, S. and Steele, R. (2002). Repressive adaptive style in children with chronic illness. *Psychosomatic Medicine.* 64 (1), 34-42.

Puchalski, C.M. (1999). FICA: A spiritual assessment. *Journal of Palliative Care,* 2-4.

Shelton, S.F., Linfield, K., Carter, B., and Morton, R (2005). Spirituality and coping with chronic life-threatening pediatric illness: Cystic fibrosis and severe asthma. *Proceedings of the American Thoracic Society (PATS),* Volume 2, Abstract Issue, 520.

Stearns, S.D., Smith, C.A., and Carter, B.D. (2000). Psychological ramifications of pediatric pain. *Clinical Pediatric Emergency Medicine,* 1 (5), 299-305.

Stewart, J.L. (2003). Children living with chronic illness: An examination of their stressors, coping responses, and health outcomes. *Annual Review of Nursing Research.* 21, 203-43.

Taylor, W.R. and Newacheck, P.W. (1992). Impact of childhood asthma on health. *Pediatrics,* 90, 657–662.

Thompson, R. J., and Gustafson, K. E. (1996). *Adaptation to chronic childhood illness.* Washington, DC: American Psychological Association.

Thompson, R.J., Gustafson, K.E., Gil, K.M., Godfrey. J., and Murphy, L.M. (1998). Illness specific patterns of psychological adjustment and cognitive adaptational processes in children with cystic fibrosis and sickle cell disease. *Journal of Clinical Psychology,* 54, 121-128.

Tix, A.P., Frazier, P.A. (1998). The use of religious coping during stressful life events main effects, moderation, and mediation. *Journal of Consulting and Clinical Psychology,* 66, 411-422.

Worthington, E.L., Kurusu, T.A., McCullough, M.E., Sandage, S.J. (1996). Empirical research on religion and psychotherapeutic processes and outcomes: A 10-year review and research prospectus. *Psychological Bulletin,* 119, 448-487.

Ziegler, J. (1998). Spirituality returns to the fold in medical practice. *Journal of the National Cancer Institute,* 90 (17), 1255-1257.

In: Religion and Healthcare   ISBN 978-1-61324-256-8
Editors: A.M. Curtis and D.P. Werthel   © 2012 Nova Science Publishers, Inc.

Chapter 5

SOME IMPLICATIONS OF INTEGRATIVE HEALTH CARE FOR RELIGION, PSYCHOLOGY AND THE HUMANITIES

Michael H. Cohen[*]

Harvard Medical School, Boston, U.S.A.

ABSTRACT

The movement to integrate complementary and alternative medical (CAM) therapies—such as acupuncture and traditional oriental medicine, chiropractic, massage therapy, and herbal medicine—into conventional health care is replete with social, ethical, institutional, and legal challenges. Overall, inclusion of CAM therapies represents a historical shift from biomedical dominance to a more inclusive, pluralistic, and holistic method of care, one that explicitly acknowledges value in healing traditions other than that variously known as "conventional care" or "biomedicine." But this movement—broadly known in some circles as "integrative medicine" (or integrative health care)—has even deeper implications than achieving a fuller range of health care choices and a more holistic model of health. Notably, with its explicit emphasis on medical pluralism, integrative health care gives voice to a broad range of healing traditions and thus weaves in insights about human health and

---

[*] Assistant Clinical Professor of Medicine, Harvard Medical School; Visiting Professor, College of the Bahamas; President, Institute for Integrative and Energy Medicine; and Principal, Law Offices of Michael H. Cohen.

healing from other disciplines. In particular, therapies relying on human consciousness and intentionality (for example, prayer, visualization, and mental healing) can be see to lie at the "borderland of healing and medicine," and thus, in the quest for understanding, to call for participation of sociologists, transpersonal psychologists, scholars of religion, and allied disciplines within the humanities. This chapter explores in preliminary form some of these links between integrative health care and religion, psychology and the humanities.

INTRODUCTION

The movement to integrate complementary and alternative medical (CAM) therapies—such as acupuncture and traditional oriental medicine, chiropractic, massage therapy, and herbal medicine—into conventional health care is replete with challenges. These include challenges to prevailing social [Ruggie, 2004], ethical [Adams, et al., 2002], institutional [Cohen and Ruggie, *Integrating*, 2004; Cohen and Ruggie, *Overcoming*, 2004], and legal [Cohen, 1998] models of health. Overall, inclusion of CAM therapies represents a historical shift from biomedical dominance to a more inclusive, pluralistic, and holistic method of care, one that explicitly acknowledges value in healing traditions other than that variously known as "conventional care" or "biomedicine" [Cohen, 1998; Cohen, 2000]. This shift also suggests a movement away from paternalism in health care and toward deeper emphasis on the ethical value of autonomy, which honors the patient's right to make decisions concerning his or her own body [Cohen, 1998].

But this movement—broadly known in some circles as "integrative medicine" (or integrative health care)—has even deeper implications than achieving a fuller range of health care choices and a more holistic model of health. Notably, with its explicit emphasis on medical pluralism, integrative health care gives voice to a broad range of healing traditions and thus weaves in insights about human health and healing from other disciplines. Indeed, a large portion of integrative health care includes therapies based on worldviews that acknowledge the role of unseen yet felt forces, such as *chi* in acupuncture and traditional oriental medicine; collectively, these therapies as "energy medicine," because they explain illness and healing in terms encompassing some notion of spiritual current or energy. Such therapies are unified in their use of diagnostic and therapeutic systems "based on the use of human consciousness and intentionality (for example, prayer, visualization, and mental healing) [Cohen 2000, *Beyond Complementary Medicine*, at 4]. They can be see to lie at the "borderland of healing and medicine" [Cohen, *Borderland*, 2004], and thus, in the quest for understanding, to call for participation of sociologists, transpersonal psychologists, scholars of religion, and allied disciplines within the humanities.

This chapter explores in preliminary form some of these links between integrative health care and religion, psychology and the humanities.

SALIENT ETHICAL VALUES

In 2005, at the conclusion of a one-year study panel, the Institute of Medicine released a report on Complementary and Alternative Medicine [IOM, 2005].[+] This Report offers a fitting opening into the implications of integrative care for religion, psychology and the humanities, because in addition to covering the bases regarding evidence-based medicine, the Report also quotes Abraham Maslow, among others (including Robert Thurman, Plato, Mary Baker Eddy, and Frieda Fromm-Reich), in an attempt to manifest the pluralistic framework and begin bridging the "conventional" and "complementary" healing arts.

While other chapters cover such topics as the state of the evidence regarding CAM therapies, gaps in evidence, research methods, education regarding CAM therapies, and models for integration, Chapter Six is entitled, *An Ethical Framework for CAM Research, Practice, and Policy*.

This chapter states that, "five major ethical commitments must be embraced," and that such ethical commitments "presuppositions or premises ... to a fair and comprehensive understanding of CAM therapies" (p. 168). The five ethical commitments (or values) are:

1. the duty of beneficence,
2. the duty of non-maleficence,
3. respect for patient autonomy,
4. recognition of medical pluralism, and
5. public accountability.

While the first three may be familiar to medical ethics, the Report frames these values in terms that heighten the commitment to expanding a sense of

[+] The author served as Consultant to the Committee on Use of Complementary and Alternative Medicine by the American Public (2004-2005) and participated in drafting the Report.

openness regarding the potential of divergent modalities to facilitate healing. For example, the first commitment includes "respecting divergent cultural beliefs; creating an emotionally safe environment for discussion of CAM; and appreciating how CAM may fit into a patient's larger social, familial, or spiritual life" (id., p. 169). Similarly, autonomy is not only respect for a specific patient's interest in making choices regarding his or her own body, but also is defined "in social terms" as "a commitment to consumer choice in health care" (id.)

The fourth and fifth commitments expand the value package. Thus, pluralism "means acknowledgement of multiple valid modes of healing and a pluralistic foundation for health care" (id.) Such acknowledgement is deemed appropriate even if some CAM practices are "rooted, at least in part, in forms of evidence and logic other than used in biomedical sciences, often with long traditions and theoretical systems of interpretation divergent from those used in biomedicine" (id.)

As to public accountability, the chapter observes that some CAM therapies "may have less kinship with technologically oriented, biomedical interventions and greater kinship with therapies at the borderland of psychological and spiritual care that are offered in professions such as pastoral counseling and hospice" (id., p. 172).

The chapter also observes that the "meaning and aim" of "integration" of CAM therapies into conventional care requires clarity around "value assumptions," as well as "negotiation about the epistemic and political assumptions" inherent in the notion of integration (id., p. 183).

And finally, while acknowledging that the "ethical principles that guide conventional biomedical research should also be applied to CAM research (id., p. 8), the Report also observes that:

> The integration of CAM therapies with conventional medicine requires that practitioners and researchers be open to diverse interpretations of health and healing, to finding innovative ways of obtaining the evidence, and to expanding the medical knowledge base (id.)

Notably, the composition of the committee that drafted the Report included an anthropologist, a clinical psychologist, a massage therapist, a licensed acupuncturist, and an ethicist, and together with medical doctors.

THE ETHICS OF INTEGRATIVE AND ENERGY MEDICINE

The Ethics chapter in the Institute of Medicine report served as a doorway to draw deeper connections between the scientific concerns of the biomedical community on one hand, and the humanistic concerns of nonmedical disciplines on the other. Put another way, ethics offered a kind of mediating force between scientific skepticism—and the demands of evidence-based approaches to medical discourse, and the inalienable logic of the human heart and spirit.

Whereas in the past, some segments of the biomedical community tended to dismiss the latter as 'irrational,' 'illogical,' and the counterparts 'non-conventional,' 'unorthodox,' and of course, 'alternative,' the Report—issued by a mainstream (and highly respected) medical authority embraced, or at least attempted to bridge, the epistemological contradictions between biomedicine and conventional. Planting its flag in the soil of "one standard" (to be applied across the board, whether a therapy is labeled "conventional" or "complementary"), the Report explicitly cautioned against "cooptation of CAM therapies by conventional medical practices" (p. 170), and softened the historic, rhetorical divide between the two camps through its references to pluralism.

From my perspective as a participant in the committee process,^ this doorway served several purposes: it softened a historical divide, to be sure; but the appearance of Maslow and the language of pluralism and accountability also formed a new bridge between the science of integrative health care, and psychology, religion, and the humanities. Thus:

> [T]he significance of a given therapeutic intervention may be less about efficacy on the physiological level and more about emotional health, coping, psychological growth, transformation, and self-actualization (Maslow, 1968).~ Likewise, therapeutic efficacy may involve such arguably vague but no less powerful spiritual themes as reconciliation with the divine or other formulations of "at-one-ment" and wholeness, or simply, perhaps, a renewed

---

^ The author apologizes for the unexpected intrusion of the subjective *I* into the objective narrative; however, the author is a human being and maintains that Heisenberg's Uncertainty Principle precludes a fully objective account. At the same time, the author's personal out-of-body explorations do suggest a possible "Witness" state of consciousness in which objectivity is possible in the sense of moving beyond the limited personality and ego.

~ Maslow AH. 1968. *Toward a Psychology of Being.* 2d ed. Princeton, NJ: Van Nostrand: Van Nostrand Insight Books.

or more expanded sense of self (Astin and Astin, 2002).⁓ Stated in these terms, providers offering (and clients availing themselves of) some of these therapies may focus less on the kind of physiological results validated by evidence in medicine and public health and more on intangible, yet nonetheless compelling, personal benefits. Such services may have less kinship with technologically oriented, biomedical interventions and greater kinship with therapies at the borderland of psychological and spiritual care that are offered in professions such as pastoral counseling and hospice.

Stated slightly differently, by virtue of their overtly psychological or spiritual aspirations, some of these therapies may have less to do with outer results and may have more to do with a kind of "inner revolution." For example, Robert Thurman links inner spiritual evolution and outer social change through Tibetan Buddhist psychological and religious teachings (Thurman, 1998). In the Western traditions, philosophers and religious thinkers as diverse as Plato and Mary Baker Eddy have ascribed to linkages between health and various ritual practices, beliefs, or ways of thinking. [IOM, p. 172 (emphasis added)]

The language of psychology, religion and spirituality appears explicitly alongside that of medicine in attempting to fathom the meaning of illness and the meaning of healing.

And the ethics chapter goes still further in bridging integrative "medicine" and the other branches of the humanities that also deal with medicine in its broadest sense:

> Thus, although physicians or public health professionals may speak in terms of morbidity, mortality, and risk factors, other kinds of clinicians and therapists may think in terms of healing the shadow self and increasing the capacity for intimacy and mature love (Fromm-Reichmann, 1960) or the growth of (and care for) the soul (Ingerman, 1991). Some physicians would even link these two domains (Ornish, 1998). In other words, public accountability, like medical pluralism, must include some consideration of the vast array of perspectives that constitute the national (and even international) heritage of healing traditions. [Id. (emphasis added)].

There is not only the soaring language referencing our planetary "heritage of healing traditions," but even room for "the soul." The whole orchestra is potentiated, not just the string or drum section—everything from soul matters to "intimacy" and even acknowledgement of the "shadow self."

⁓ Astin JA, Astin AW. 2002. An integral approach to medicine. *Alternative Therapies in Health & Medicine* 8(2):70–75.

And it is entirely appropriate that the profession of medicine—together with allied and complementary care professions, and now aided by scholars of religion and psychology and other disciplines—scale the heights of healing and encompass all the light and darkness, from mature love, intimacy, and soul contact to healing the shadow aspects of being.

THE FARTHER REACHES

My own interest in spirituality and healing is not accidental.

A short version of a longer memoir [Cohen, *Friends*, 2005] is necessary to explain. I had always been interested in psychology and religion, having been steeped in Torah, Talmud, and Jewish learning through childhood. In college, I pursued a rational, left-brain course, studying political science and international affairs. In fact, I wrote my college thesis on nuclear deterrence strategy. One could fairly say my emotional life was undeveloped, or lacked a full container for satisfactory expression. I did not turn to drugs or crime— rather, I sublimated. Meanwhile, though, I began having out-of-body experience in my dorm room at Columbia University. I could not explain these sensations of paralysis, floating above my body, and the like—and the explanation of "generalized anxiety" and reduction of mystical experience to "symptoms" did not satisfy. To appease my intellectual curiosity, I read Jung, and flung my body about various dance clubs to express the "Dionysian frenzy" inside.

After graduating law school with sufficient academic standing to enter a top Wall Street firm, I first spent a year serving as a law clerk to a federal judge in New York. That year confirmed my reservations about the power of law alone (embodying the archetype of Reason) to achieve justice. There seemed to be little room for the emotions—alternatively, they were compressed into the boundaries and artifices of legal language and procedure.

The year after the clerkship, I returned to business school, and then spent a third year (and a half) at the Iowa Writers Workshop. I was lucky to be accepted; and felt that perhaps in creative writing I might find a way to more fully express my spirit than through law. There was emotion aplenty at the Workshop, expressed through fiction, poetry, and everyday exchange—some capable of transporting me to inner heights, and much of the narcissism, insecurity, and pettiness that also characterizes individuals within a competitive community trying to emerge as artists. Neither the potion nor its antidote brought resolution to the inner conflicts that increasingly manifested in dreams and creative writing; could I find a third way?

I eventually found works of Georges I. Gurdjieff and P.D. Ouspensky explicating and advocating exactly that—or something a bit more advanced, a fourth way, *the* Third Way, they called it, perhaps to emphasis its transcendental and unique authority. The tools of what Gurdjieff called "self-observation" and "self-remembering" marked efforts to attain greater clarity of consciousness than the whipsaw of mental reasoning and the emotions. Then, in Iowa City, I encountered various ex-patriots among the would-be literati and began practicing yoga and meditating. A great shift in awareness occurred—suddenly I was reading works by Charles Tart and others on altered states of consciousness, exploring lucid dreaming, and realizing that the life of my unconscious was far greater than I had supposed.

As Milton H. Erickson, MD used to put it:

> "Your conscious mind is very intelligent... but your unconscious mind is a lot smarter... and so I'm not asking you to learn any new skills... I'm only asking you to be willing to utilize the skills you already have, but do not yet fully know about." [Gilligan, p. 72]

Or, as a hypnotherapy instructor paraphrased:

> *Your conscious mind is very intelligent, but your unconscious mind is a whole lot smarter. So why not let it do the work for a change?*

Very Ericksonian—"let it do the work for a change." My unconscious was dreaming me. Turning to my political science roots for a metaphor, James Madison had written this:

> If men were angels, no government would be necessary. If angels were to govern men, neither external nor internal controls on government would be necessary.[**]

Clearly there was a state in which I could partake of both the human and the angelic, and then attempt a kind of self psycho-synthesis, bridging the

---

[**] Madison continued with this: "In framing a government which is to be administered by men over men, the great difficulty lies in this: you must first enable the government to control the governed; and in the next place oblige it to control itself." James Madison, The Federalist No. 51.

various spiritual disciplines and teachings within me, and then drawing on this unity to do my work in the world.

Pluralism has spawned from within.

THE POSSIBLE PARAMETERS OF HEALING

From the personal to the impersonal (and back again), the journey continues. In *Beyond Complementary Medicine*, I noted that the literature to date had drawn a distinction between "curing" and "healing." For example, curing, for example, might involve treating breast cancer through radical lumpectomy, while healing might involve addressing underlying or accompanying psycho-spiritual issues; thus, a patient could be cured without being healed, and conversely healed without being cured.

The distinction between curing and healing had some utility—the former generally thought to be the province of biomedicine, the latter that of CAM modalities such as those involving energy healing. And there are legal implications in terms of scope of practice, medical doctors being assigned by their licensure the entire province of alleviating disease, and all other providers relegated to a specified subset of this sphere [Cohen, 1998].

But over time, the goal of integration has suggested a blending of these goals. At its best, beside medicine aim to be (and can be) healing; and CAM therapies purport to have curative value (hence the emphasis on finding a satisfactory evidentiary base for the integration of these therapies). In *Beyond Complementary Medicine*, I defined "healing" as "moving toward wholeness at all levels of being," suggesting that this definition "can and should force Western culture to reexamine its assumptions about life and consciousness" [Cohen, *Beyond* 2000, at 142]. I also suggested that expressing the definition in this way "challenges a health care system that views pathology largely in material terms, that defines scientific truth in biophysical realities, that dismisses the 'irrational' and the 'mystical'" [id., at 144-145]. In the chapter on bioethics, I juxtaposed inner experience with analysis in order "to validate subjectivity, intuition, and mystery in equipoise to science and law" [id.].

Beyond Complementary Medicine suggested that rather than viewing CAM therapies and providers through the sole lens of preventing fraud (a frequent rationale in legislative history and judicial decision-making concerning such therapies and providers), the legal paradigm ought to consider other perspectives and values [p. 19]. These included not only quality assurance (the attempt to ensure competence), but also health care freedom (principally the autonomy value), functional integration of medical systems (the pluralism principle), and finally, the possibility for achieving human transformation through one or more therapies. I noted that both individual and social transformation stood at the apex of a "hierarchy of values governing medicine:"

> Just as the evolution of the human being and humanity toward the Godhead (known in some traditions as God-realization, enlightenment, the Christ Self, or the Buddha nature) is an explicit objective in the spiritual technologies used in energy healing ... similarly, the goal of transformation supports an evolutionary process within the legal and regulatory framework. Id.

In other words, the power of law could be used to shape and guide the possible parameters of healing. Law was a tool not only for curbing fraud, but also for facilitating transformation—however that term might be defined through the lens of religion, psychology, and the humanities.

Thus the dots were connected: law and ethics in complementary, alternative, and integrative medicine led explicitly to what Maslow termed "the farther reaches of human nature" and to illumination of mystical experience, alternative states of consciousness, and inner realities through these disciplines outside of, yet potently cousin to, both biomedicine and CAM.

MOVING TOWARD WHOLENESS AT ALL LEVELS OF BEING

Future Medicine [Cohen, *Future Medicine*, 2003] went further and explicitly analogized Maslow's famous hierarchy of needs, to a hypothetical *regulatory* hierarchy of needs. Maslow, as we know, described five sets of basic needs in the following ascending hierarchy [Maslow, 1968]:

1. *Physiological*: These include the need for food; sleep; various sensory pleasures (such as tastes, smells, stroking).
2. *Safety*: These include the need for security; stability; dependency; protection; freedom from fear, anxiety and chaos; structure, order, law, and limits; and strength in the protector.
3. *Belongingness and love*: These include the need for relationships and for giving and receiving affection.

4. *Esteem*: These include the desire for achievement, adequacy, mastery and competence, independence and freedom, as well as for reputation, status, recognition, dignity, and appreciation.
5. *Self- actualization*: This involves the need to do what the individual is fitted for; being true to one's nature; being self-fulfilled, or actualized in what the person is potentially.

Maslow also argued that while these needs were constantly coming to the background and then foreground of human experience, a complete human was one who managed to satisfy all five sets of needs; and further, that a person thwarted in *any* of the basic needs was sick or at least less than fully alive (id.). He rejected a theory of motivation based on neurosis, and instead urged a theory building on the highest capacities of health, including self-actualization and the capacity for what he termed "peak experiences," clear realizations of ultimate goodness, capacity, and radiance on all levels.

Future Medicine drew a parallel between each level of needs and corresponding regulatory objectives. Thus, the regulatory objective of fraud control—which tends to dominate legal impulse over health care—corresponds with physiological needs, in its effort to address the base-level survival struggles of humane experience. The next level up the hierarchy is quality assurance, which roughly corresponds with the personal need to achieve safety.

The third value, that of health care freedom, corresponds with Maslow's articulation of belongingness in community, as health care patients and consumers can only truly "belong" once they feel in charge of decisions concerning their own bodily health. The fourth, the esteem need, is met by granting respect to the world's healing traditions—not judging, dismissing, or arbitrarily condemning, but rather according esteem to divergent world traditions and philosophies concerning human health and healing. Fifth and finally, self-actualization corresponds with the regulatory goal of transformation, as encouraging the peak of human experience is the explicit goal of many CAM therapies (notably some hands-on spiritual healing therapies, as well as meditation and prayer—to the extent the latter is included in typologies of CAM therapies) and frequently becomes a facet of even conventional medicine (as in counseling accompanying end-of-life care).

Following Maslow's argument, *Future Medicine* urged that at any given time, one or more of these various regulatory values may come to the foreground—fraud control and transformation, for example, both are important; one need not necessarily be sacrificed or discarded for the other.

The question is the extent to which the regulatory structure will reflect all five values, or continue a narrow focus on fraud control (and sometimes quality assurance).

More to the point, in the absence of input from psychology, religion, and other disciplines in the humanities, the (sometimes) parochial language of biomedicine can exclude the farther reaches of the hierarchy of both human and social/regulatory needs. Dismissing all CAM therapies as 'unproven' or 'unethical,' for example—or using language such as "quackery" (recall the American Medical Association's Committee on Quackery, which was successfully challenged in *Wilk v. AMA*)—presumes that all non-biomedical healers require fraud control and leave no room to offer transcendence. Contrast for a moment the Buddhist practice of *tonglen*, which breathes in a person's suffering and breathes out compassion, and offers a more transpersonal (and holistic) approach to, say, intensive care than relegating all ritual to fanciful (subjective and hence indeterminate) religious practice.

Maslow characterized as sick a motivational theory directed only to the misdirection of neurotics; similarly, a regulatory structure that focuses on fraud control to the exclusion of acknowledging the possibility for transcendence is weak and flawed, and under-serves patients in need of care at all levels of being. If medicine is also a ministry (as biomedical physicians in the best tradition of medicine have urged) then transcendence has a place not only in integrative health care, but also in its component branches. The implications for rethinking health care law and policy are vast (see *Future Medicine* for a beginning contemplation), but essentially, the notion is that aligning some of the work done in psychology (beginning with Maslow) with new thinking regarding regulation of CAM therapies opens the door to new insights than the usual debates about where, why, and how we want to create rules governing clinical and institutional provision of, and patient access to, a full spectrum of therapeutic modalities.

And ultimately, discussion of law and policy lead from the base of the pyramid to its apex, and hence to a conversation about the role of health—in its broadest sense (including self-actualization and transformation)—care, and this ongoing process called human (spiritual) evolution.

THE HUMAN ENERGY FIELD AND BEYOND

The need to bridge integrative health care and the humanities is just beginning to receive recognition in the literature, notably in an edited volume entitled *The role of complementary and alternative medicine: accommodating pluralism* [Callahan, 1996].

What if the human being is more than the body, and luminous filaments can be traced that connect human beings not only to each other, but also to larger universal forces? What if the archetypes are not only psychological stuff, existing inside the head (or projected in the white screen of the mind onto others) but living entities, existing inter-dimensionally in spectrums of consciousness observable to consciousness, but currently difficult to measure through objectively cognizable instrumentation? Yet, what if energy medicine research (and work in physics, mathematics, and other disciplines) are beginning to validate the existence of these other realms of existence, heretofore described only by religious traditions and the 'soft' science of psychology? What if possibilities for human consciousness are far greater than imagined, and a certain unity among religious traditions (as asserted by many mystics) traces a path to a spiritual technology as, or more potent, than electro-mechanical-biochemical pathways currently known and acknow-ledged?

And what if the contemplatively revealed answers to these questions (and successive labyrinths of revelation) require altering our fundamental thinking about what we want to accomplish through regulation? Might we find, by exploring the farther reaches of human nature, what lies at the ultimate end of the road of consciousness, that we no longer need regulate solely out of fear and need to control the Shadow, but can actually converse with the Wise Old Person of myth within? How would law, public policy, ethics, and regulation have to adapt to changing notions of what a human being is?

Energy healing posits that a human beings stands within a human energy field (HEF)—the term *aura* is used within a more spiritual vein, although the HEF, an acronym, gives a more scientific flavor. No researcher, however, has been able to identify exactly what the "energy" is, and energy is an awkward term (the Chantilly Report, a 1992 report to the Office of Alternative Medicine at the National Institutes of Medicine, preferred the term "biofield therapeutics," which is not much in use, and the National Center for Complementary and Alternative Medicine now speaks of "frontier medicine") [Chantilly Report]. Nonetheless, no substitute terminology has emerged. In any event, the egg-shaped aura can be perceived with a modicum of training, even though there is scientific controversy about whether it exists and can be measured—or at least can be validated through measurement of its effects [Jonas and Crawford, 2003].

From a legal perspective based on contemporary legal rules, *Future Medicine* suggested that the emergence of energy healing presents at least four emerging regulatory conundrums: first, whether and how to license providers practicing some form of energy healing; second, how to define healers' scope of practice; third, establishing a standard of care, for purposes of determining the boundaries of acceptable practice; fourth, appropriate documentation of the application of energy healing. Yet, moving even beyond these present legal conundrums, legal rules pertaining to health care historically have followed the assumptions of biomedicine that the human being is identified with the body, and that anything beyond that is "religious" and hence inaccessible to medicine [Cohen, *Borderland*, 2005]. A patient's religious perspectives can and even should be acknowledged, but the law itself cannot and does not intrude into religious questions (such as whether life extends beyond the body).

This dilemma leads to some very difficult choices—and awkward philosophical distinctions; for example, it is frequently considered unethical (and illegal) to practice *active euthanasia*—to affirmatively provide a dying patient who is in terrible pain with a substance that will expedite the dying; yet, ethical (and legal) to practice *passive euthanasia*—such as starving the body to death by withholding nutrition and hydration. Of course, there are good and valid reasons for these philosophical distinctions—among them the difficult in drawing limits once active euthanasia is allowed; yet, what is ultimately considered ethical and legal may be divorced from what might be considered compassionate. Put rhetorically, is it better to starve someone to death or to ease them gently into that great transition, using a combination of substances and ritual to help clear and illuminate the mind during the dying?

One might consider this an "integrative health care" approach to dying. From a more conventional standpoint, the notion of the "good death" or "peaceful death" is gaining currency in bioethical literature; yet still, because biomedicine and the law that governs it cannot pry beyond the physical veil—this is the province of religion—dilemmas persist.

And these dilemmas persist in every sector of bioethics. *Future Medicine* briefly addresses dying, and reproductive technologies—two ends of the spectrum of life—and suggests that views of consciousness from psychology and religion may greatly inform biomedical, bioethical, and legal perspectives. If hypnotherapy, guided imagery, and the healer's own intuitive perception can help guide a dying person, and some consensus (beyond warring beliefs) can someday be drawn regarding the mystical experience of dying (incorporating, perhaps, the literature on near-death and out-of-body experiences), perhaps such literature can inform institutional protocol, as well as liability and ethical concerns of clinicians involved.

As Beyond Complementary Medicine argued (p. 77):

> Yet another area of potential contribution–or stimulus and provocation–from practitioners of energy healing involves medical ethics, particularly at the boundaries of birth and death. Whereas Western medicine, and thus bioethics, tends to split science and religion, energy healing regards sentient beings, from animals to patients in a "persistent vegetative state," as having consciousness on some level--irrespective of whether such consciousness can be measured through medical concepts and instruments. Because secular humanism regards attempts to describe consciousness, outside of medical measurement, as speculative and futile, Western medicine and medical ethics frequently strive to perpetuate biological existence at all costs; to draw artificial boundaries between life and death; and to assume that animals, pre-embryos (who can be "selectively terminated"), anencephalic infants (who are born without a brainstem thus presumed to have only a reflexive response to painful stimuli), and other life forms lack consciousness, or do not deserve our respect and freedom from undue or undignified invasion. As discussed in Chapters 10 through 12, perspectives from energy healing can enrich and inform such topics as multifetal pregnancy reduction, decisions regarding termination of life support, and organ donation.

A pluralistic perspective has much to offer contemporary bioethics, particularly if 'non-ordinary' states of consciousness can inform debates that are typically framed in dualistic terms (e.g., legal/illegal, permissible /impermissible, ethical/unethical).

And *Future Medicine* provocatively asked:

> Might some medical orders be contraindicated on a spiritual level, and how can this [spiritual] information be integrated into a medical system that does not—yet—incorporate spiritual perspectives so as to explicitly acknowledge these dimensions of being?

Future bioethics might incorporate "such premises as, for instance, the notion that relationships between living and dead persons are important," or the suggestion "that apprehension of such relationships might be gleaned through such therapies as hypnosis and guided imagery, homeopathy, and energy healing."

One of the experiences reported in *Beyond Complementary Medicine* involved a client in a healing practice who had had an abortion. The healer^^^ did not know of this history, but during the healing opened to an altered state of consciousness and perceived a being, in the form of a fragmented fetus, in the client's energy field. During the healing, the author telepathically connected with both the client and the fetus and facilitated a therapeutic conversation between the two.

This is obviously not the kind of case study necessarily that would be published in mainstream medical journal. And, for reasons having more to do with accepted epistemologies than intellectual rigor, revealing this kind of an experience to a psychotherapist could be fraught with peril. And yet, if a human being is more than the body, than bioethical frameworks may benefit from conversation from such perspectives.

The question of the soul—raised in the Institute of Medicine chapter on ethics—recurs again and again. Although the veil of the material may, at this point, preclude the kind of objective scientific investigation and validation that makes us comfortable, still, consensus mystical experience may yield insights in terms of penetrating beyond the veil of what Charles Tart has called "consensus trance" [Tart, 1986].

CONCLUSION

Integrative health care reflects a new movement in clinicians' and institutions' attempts to combine biomedical (conventional) care and CAM therapies to create the best menu of options for the patient. Debates around integrative care thus far largely have occurred in medical literature, centering on questions of safety and efficacy. It is now time to more deeply explore the emerging connections between holistic, pluralistic, and integrative models of care with insights into health and healing from religion, psychology, and the humanities.

---

^^^ The author.

ACKNOWLEDGMENTS

The author acknowledges with gratitude support for this work from the Frederick S. Upton Foundation and the Helen M. and Annetta E. Himmelfarb Foundation. The author also appreciates the special efforts of Larry Mervine, Professor Sherman Cohn of Georgetown University, and David S. Upton.

REFERENCES

Adams KE, Cohen MH, Jonsen AR, Eisenberg DM. (2002) Ethical considerations of complementary and alternative medical therapies in conventional medical settings. Ann Intern Med; 137: 660-664.

Alternative Medicine: Expanding Medical Horizons (A Report to the National Institutes of Health on Alternative Medical Systems and Practices in the United States), 134-142 (September 14-16, 1992) (the Chantilly Report).

Callahan Daniel, (2002) The role of complementary and alternative medicine: accommodating pluralism.; Washington, D.C.: Georgetown University Press.

Cohen MH. A friend of all faiths. 2005; Mutton Fish Point Publishing.

Cohen MH. Beyond complementary medicine: legal and ethical perspectives on health care and human evolution. Ann Arbor: University of Michigan Press; 2000.

Cohen MH. (1998) Complementary and alternative medicine: legal boundaries and regulatory perspectives. Baltimore: Johns Hopkins University Press; 180 pages.

Cohen MH. (2003) Future medicine: ethical dilemmas, regulatory challenges, and therapeutic pathways to health and healing in human transformation. Ann Arbor: University of Michigan Press; 350 pages.

Cohen MH. Healing at the borderland of medicine and religion: regulating potential abuse of authority by spiritual healers. 18:2 J Law and Relig 2004;373-426.

Cohen MH, Ruggie M. (2004) Integrating complementary and alternative medical therapies in conventional medical settings: legal quandaries and potential policy models. Cinn L Rev; 72:2: 671-729.

Cohen MH, Ruggie M. (2004) Overcoming legal and social barriers to integrative medicine. Medical Law Intl 6: 339-393.

Ernst EE, Cohen MH. (2001) Informed consent in complementary and alternative medicine. Arch Intern Med;161:19: 2288-2292.

Ernst EE, Cohen MH, Stone J. (2004) Ethical problems arising in evidence-based complementary and alternative medicine. J Med Ethics;30: 156-159.

Gilligan Stephen G, Therapeutic trances (New York: Brunner/Mazel, 1987).

Healing, Intention and Energy Medicine (Wayne B. Jonas and Cindy C. Crawford, eds.) (New York: Churchill Livingstone, 2003).

Institute of Medicine of the National Academies of Science, Complementary and Alternative Medicine (Washington, D.C.: National Academies Press, 2005).

Ruggie, M. (2004) Marginal to mainstream: alternative medicine in America. Cambridge: Cambridge Univ. Press.

Tart, C. Waking up: overcoming the obstacles to human potential. Boston: New Science Library, 1986.

INDEX

D

Hispanics, 94
historical data, 34
history, 16, 115, 122
holism, 14, 19, 21, 29, 42
holistic care, 14, 19, 39, 46, 60
honesty, 19
hope, 75
hopelessness, 20
hospice, 110, 112
hospitalization, 30, 33, 34, 36, 46, 48, 49, 96
hostility, 44
housing, 72, 73, 77
human, ix, 2, 14, 15, 16, 17, 19, 20, 22, 29, 38, 39, 46, 48, 49, 50, 52, 53, 54, 55, 58, 60, 62, 63, 86, 104, 107, 108, 111, 114, 116, 117, 118, 119, 120, 122, 123, 124
human condition, 15
human development, 104
human dimensions, 14
human experience, 15, 17, 53, 117
human health, ix, 14, 107, 108, 117
human nature, 116, 119
human sciences, 62
humanism, 17, 61, 121
humanistic nursing, viii, 13, 16, 17, 18, 46, 49, 57, 58, 59
Hunter, 6, 7
hyperactivity, 94, 96
hypnosis, 121
hypnotherapy, 114, 120
hypothesis, 23, 95

I

ideal, 6
ideals, 29
ideas, 18
identity, 35, 87, 92
illumination, 116
image, 2, 54
imagery, 120, 121
imagination, 19
immortality, 54, 60
immune system, 57, 84

implementation, 58
improvements, 90
inclusion, ix, 107, 108
income, 75, 87
independence, 117
indication, 23
indicators, 21, 61
indices, 94, 96
individual, 72, 73, 74, 75, 76, 77
individuality, 49
individualization, 26, 50
individuals, 5, 6, 7, 8, 10, 16, 17, 20, 21, 29, 37, 48, 53, 58, 66, 75, 84, 92, 113
individuation, 74
industries, 30
inequality, 3
infants, 121
influence, viii, 13, 85, 86, 87, 92, 93, 96, 101, 105
injury, viii, 81
input, 44, 118
insecurity, 113
insight, 21, 29, 42
institutions, 56, 122
instruction, 50
instruments, 121
insulin, 104
insulin dependent diabetes, 104
integration, 59, 66, 78, 89, 109, 110, 115, 116
integrity, 88
intensity, 85
intent, 18
intentionality, ix, 108
interaction, 20, 36, 50, 52
interactions, 26, 61
interest, viii, 15, 34, 81, 82, 84, 94, 101, 110, 113
internal controls, 114
internalizing, 94, 95
international affairs, 113
interpretation, 17, 61, 95, 96, 110
intervention, 20, 86, 89, 100, 101, 111
interventions, 66, 69